W9-AWM-927

green baby

Susannah Marriott

Consultant Editor Lawrence Rosen, MD

LONDON, NEW YORK, MELBOURNE, MUNICH, and DELHI

Y'n gweras yma'n gorthyp
(A Cornish saying: In the soil lies the answer)

US editor Christine Heilman
Project editor Tara Woolnough
Designer Hannah Moore
Project art editor Sara Kimmins
Photographer Tim Evan-Cook
Illustrator Anna Hymas
Managing editors Esther Ripley, Penny Warren
Managing art editor Marianne Markham
Jacket concept Sophia Tampakopoulos, Bryn Walls
Jacket designer Peggy Sadler
Production editor Ben Marcus
Production controller Wendy Penn
Creative technical support Sonia Charbonnier
Category publisher Peggy Vance

First American Edition, 2008

Published in the United States by
DK Publishing, 375 Hudson Street, New York, New York 10014

08 09 10 11   10 9 8 7 6 5 4 3 2 1
GD112—June 2008

Published in Great Britain by Dorling Kindersley Limited.

A catalog record for this book is available from the Library of Congress.
ISBN 978-0-7566-3673-9

DK books are available at special discounts when purchased in bulk for sales promotions, premiums,
fund-raising, or educational use. For details, contact: DK Publishing Special Markets, 375 Hudson
Street, New York, New York 10014 or SpecialSales@dk.com.

Color reproduced in Singapore by Colourscan
Printed and bound in Germany by Mohn Media

Mixed Sources
Product group from well-managed
forests and other controlled sources
www.fsc.org Cert no. SA-COC-1592
© 1996 Forest Stewardship Council
FSC

Discover more at
www.dk.com

Foreword

Green is hot, and families across the globe are
looking for practical guidance on how to go green;
but what does it mean to have a "green baby"?

In my role as a pediatrician and medical advisor to the Deirdre
Imus Environmental Center, every day I witness the impact of
environmental changes on our children's health. The rise in rates
of allergies and asthma, cancer, obesity and diabetes, autism, and
other disorders can be traced directly to changes in our planet's
ecosystem. Our best path to wellness includes adopting the methods
detailed in this highly practical guide to green parenting. This book
takes a comprehensive look at those aspects of green living that
affect you and your children most, and explains that raising a green
baby is a lifestyle commitment to caring for your whole child, while
respecting the interaction of health and our environment. As you
embark on the important journey of parenting, you will find this
new handbook very useful; it may, in fact, change your life.

Green living is no longer simply a nice concept—it is an
absolute imperative as we seek to improve the state of our
children's health and the health of our planet, our collective
home. Our children are our most precious natural resource, and
indeed, their future is in our hands.

Lawrence D. Rosen, MD (Chair, Integrative Pediatrics Council)

Contents

INTRODUCTION

What actually is a "green" lifestyle, and
how could it make a difference for your family
and your baby, not to mention the planet?

The green agenda has become identified with climate change, carbon
dioxide being its chief culprit (see pp.9–11). But if we concentrate
only on cutting carbon emissions, we miss the bigger green picture.
This only comes into focus when we look at the kind of lifestyle that
motivates our growing carbon emissions: shopping at suburban
supermarkets with the same range of goods wherever we live;
buying disposable fashions that go out of style every five weeks;
being so busy we drive to places where we could walk to; eating out-
of-season produce from across the planet; accruing electronic goods;
and keeping a home warm enough for shorts all year-round. This life
is unsustainable, whether underpinned by green or "brown" energy.

It's quite simple to be greener. Each of us—parents and babies
alike—just needs to consume less. If we can do this, we also cut back
on some of the synthetic chemicals that sustain modern life (e.g., in
killing pests, making plastic flexible, preventing artificial objects
from becoming a fire hazard) but also pollute the only things we
really need: clean air, water, soil, food, bodies—and breast milk.
Living green also means reconnecting to the places we live; by
anchoring our lives in our local environment, from electricity to
diapers, we create a truly green place to raise our babies.

THE HEALTH OF THE PLANET

The world's climate is changing. These are facts every parent needs to know, in order to understand why we need to act now to preserve Earth.

The world's leading authority on climate change and its impact, the IPCC (Intergovernmental Panel on Climate Change), states that humans are responsible for most of the global-warming effect observed over the past 50 years, mainly by changing Earth's atmospheric gases. A number of gases (known as greenhouse gases) cause Earth to warm up: the most important is water vapor; the second, carbon dioxide (CO_2); others include methane, nitrous oxide, and ozone. Burning fossil fuels (oil, coal, and natural gas) and clearing forests are the primary human activities that have intensified this warming, since both release huge stores of carbon dioxide. What's the result? An increased likelihood of extreme weather, from torrential downpours and flooding to heat waves and "wildcat" fires; the warming of lakes, rivers, and seas; a shift in flora and fauna; and increased risk of species extinction.

Between 1970 and 2004, CO_2 emissions increased by 80%

Introduction

How might this affect the world our children will inherit? If it reduces agricultural land and biodiversity, and brings changes to the seasons and water availability, our ability to produce enough food will be seriously impaired. Heat waves may trigger changes in the distribution of infectious diseases and greater mortality. Settlements in low-lying coastal regions or flood plains and mountains may be at risk. Social and economic instability, migration, and wars could follow.

Many organisms and ecosystems will struggle to adapt to climate change

Greenhouse gas emissions rose by 70 percent between 1970 and 2004, the largest increase coming from energy supplies, closely followed by transportation. This trend is projected to continue up to 2030, as developing countries increase carbon dioxide emissions. But don't blame these countries; although it produces many of our consumer goods, the developing world's emissions are predicted to remain substantially lower than those of developed countries—in 1999 a mere eight nations were responsible for almost 50 percent of carbon dioxide emissions globally: the US, Canada, Russia, Japan, the UK, Germany, France, and Italy.

Introduction

The future of our babies is in our hands. We may have only 12–15 years to stabilize greenhouse gases: after that we may not be able to stop the juggernaut. However, the IPCC agrees that modifying lifestyle and consumption patterns can reduce emissions. Using fewer resources has a positive effect, as do measures like managing transportation and urban planning. Which way will we choose? We are the first generation to be able to take a lead, and pass on to our children the skills and technology to make life sustainable again.

Industrial consumption of natural resources and the consequent pollution have already radically altered our planet.

The basics of going green

"Reduce, reuse, and recycle" is the mantra of green parents; deep greens add in "refuse" and "repair." Notice where "recycle" comes in the list—if you do the first two, this tends to take care of itself.

The rules

- **Refuse**—you don't need most items touted in parenting magazines. Talk to parents of older babies about what they could have done without. Don't accept plastic bags or excessive packaging. Above all, refuse fossil fuels by driving less, turning down the thermostat, and buying fewer air-freighted foods.
- **Reduce**—try three rather than five sleepers; walk, don't drive; and cut back on plastic toys (they waste oil, a precious resource that keeps carbon safely tucked away underground).
- **Reuse**—reusable bags are the easiest, but try cloth diapers, hardly worn clothes, and furniture from reclaimed lumber.
- **Repair**—only allow into your home items that are built to last and that you'll want to repair and keep forever.
- **Recycle**—the last option when you can't fix something or pass it on; how do you need to recycle?

Play the recycling game with your baby and it'll be second nature by the time he's a toddler.

A perfect time to change

A new baby often means rethinking every part of life: use this impetus to start living sustainably, and teach your child great green habits for life.

In the past 20 years, humankind's environmental footprint has increased dramatically with our snowballing use of natural resources, land, and energy. How you work and travel, where you live, what you eat, and when (or if) you sleep are all up for grabs after giving birth. Start making a difference with the resources consumed on your baby's behalf. This might seem crazy at a time when you're encouraged to consume more—to buy booties, beds, and bottles—but your baby's future is a mighty motivator.

Simple green tips

- Do you need to fill the teakettle to make up a feeding? Boil only the amount of water you need.
- Are you doing more laundry now that you have reusable diapers? To reduce your impact on natural resources, replace detergent with laundry-balls and hang diapers out on the clothesline to dry.
- Do you find that you're using more tissues and toilet paper to clean up? Switch to a brand that's at least 80 percent post-consumer recycled; plant a tree or two; and join an environmental organization.

- Are you switching on the lights and heating more frequently now that you're at home more? Insulate everything you can; turn off or unplug appliances instead of leaving them on standby; and fight the urge to buy electronic baby gadgets. Ask your electric company if you can choose to buy a portion of your electricity from renewable sources.
- Another mouth to feed? Choose seasonal produce from your region (more greenhouse gases are emitted flying in food than by the air-travel industry). When you eat meat, make sure it's locally sourced and ethically raised.

Before throwing something away, first ask yourself where its ingredients came from and where they'll end up; are any hazardous for the environment? Could the item go somewhere else (for example, to a friend, or the recycling center), or could you have bought an alternative item with a longer life? If thinking this way causes you to buy less in the future, going green will make your life noticeably more streamlined, even with a baby.

During 2004–2005,
the amount of
food air-freighted
to the UK rose by 31%

Environmental impact, known as a carbon footprint, is measured in acres

In the West, our carbon footprint is now 54 acres per person. Earth's capacity is just 40 acres per person

Parental responsibilities

There's nothing like having a baby for making you more aware of your responsibilities, including not wrecking the planet for the next generation.

The human population has increased by one-third since 1987. As the standard of global living conditions also rises, so does pressure on basic resources such as water and land, as well as on biodiversity—and energy-related carbon dioxide emissions. So by creating more potential consumers of energy and resources, we parents are actually contributing to the problem!

Parents who commit to a green lifestyle, however, are doing their part to help ease the strain on our planet. They will choose to consume less overall and more ethically, avoiding products created by companies whose actions harm the environment. You can check out the environmental and ethical record of many companies by doing a little online research.

There is such an abundance of ethical, organic goods available today that more and more of us are going green: for example, we might choose to toss out our old mattresses, sofas, clothes, and cosmetics, and ship in greener versions instead. But to be responsibly green, it's important to think minimal and local. Although this can seem like an onerous responsibility, it's also a feel-good opportunity to teach children that material possessions don't really equal happiness.

Introduction

How green is your family?

Select the answers that best reflect the way you live now to find out how green your lifestyle is, and how you can become more eco-friendly.

HOME

1 Is your home well insulated?
A No; it's an old, drafty house.
B No, but we shut windows and doors, and close the curtains at dusk to keep in heat.
C Yes; our house is a qualified Energy Star home.

2 How green is your energy?
A Not at all; we leave appliances on standby all the time.
B We use energy-efficient light bulbs and appliances.
C We buy green electricity.

3 Do you recycle?
A We're not very clear about what can be recycled.
B We put out everything for a curbside collection.
C We have a compost pile and don't create much waste because we refuse, reuse, and repair things.

4 How do you save energy?
A By turning down the thermostat.
B We unplug everything when not in use.
C We got rid of our TV and turn off lights if we're not in the room.

FAMILY FOOD

1 What do you usually eat?
A Convenience food.
B Home-cooked dishes.
C Vegetarian home-cooked dishes.

2 Where do you buy most food?
A At the supermarket.
B From the local organic supermarket and health-food store.
C At the farmers' market.

3 Where do your organic fruit and vegetables come from?
A Overseas, via the supermarket.
B A CSA subscription.
C We grow our own.

4 How do you carry your shopping?
A In plastic bags from the cashier.
B In heavy-duty reusable plastic bags.
C In fair-trade cotton bags.

BABY FOOD

1 Where does your baby's milk come from?
A Regular formula.
B A combination of organic formula and breast milk.
C Breast milk.

2 If you're breastfeeding, what bodycare products do you use?
  A Whatever I find on sale.
  B Certified organic products.
  C Nothing I wouldn't eat.

3 What are your baby's first foods?
  A Store-bought purees.
  B Homemade organic purees.
  C Regular family food, mashed or cut into pieces.

4 What does your toddler eat?
  A Packaged toddler meals.
  B Mostly home-cooked organic children's food: fish sticks, pasta.
  C Whatever we're eating.

BABY CLOTHING

1 What does your baby usually wear next to his skin?
  A Sleepers from an economy pack.
  B New organic cotton, hemp, or bamboo.
  C Cotton hand-me-downs.

2 Where are your baby clothes from?
  A Manufactured in East Asia.
  B Made in the US.
  C Fair-trade projects.

3 What do you do with old clothes?
  A We throw them away.
  B Put them in with the recycling.
  C Hand them on to friends or charity.

4 How often do you wash baby clothes?
  A After each wearing.
  B When they need washing.
  C Only once we have enough for a full load, along with our regular laundry.

BABY TOYS

1 What do you use as a teether?
  A A plastic teether.
  B Organic cotton.
  C A wooden teething ring.

2 What are your soft toys made of?
  A Synthetic fabrics.
  B Organic cotton, hemp, and bamboo.
  C Fair-trade organic fabrics stuffed with untreated wool.

3 Where do you buy toys?
  A From the department store.
  B From natural baby stores, catalogs, and websites.
  C From garage sales, secondhand stores, and online auctions.

4 Does your child have any battery-operated toys?
  A Yes, many.
  B Yes, but we only use rechargeable batteries.
  C No, we prefer wooden or wind-up clockwork toys.

DIAPERS AND WIPES

1 Which type of diapers do you use?
  A Regular disposables.
  B Fully biodegradable disposables.
  C Reusable diapers.

2 How do you wash reusables?
  A At 140°F (60°C), with regular detergent and fabric conditioner.
  B At 140°F (60°C), with eco-detergent.
  C At 104°F (40°C), with laundry-balls.

3 Do you use baby wipes?
   A Yes, all the time.
   B Yes, but the organic type.
   C No, we make our own.

4 How do you deal with diaper rash?
   A With regular diaper-rash cream.
   B With certified organic cream.
   C We use homeopathic cream.

CLEANING

1 What do you wash clothes with?
   A Regular detergent.
   B Eco-detergent.
   C Laundry-balls or soap nuts.

2 How do you dry clothes?
   A In a dryer than turns itself off when clothes are dry.
   B At the laundromat.
   C We mostly line dry.

3 How do you clean surfaces?
   A With bleach-based cream cleaners.
   B With an eco-spray.
   C With lemon juice or vinegar.

4 How do you clean carpets?
   A Steam cleaning.
   B A sprinkling of bicarbonate of soda and vacuum cleaner.
   C We don't have carpets.

BABY'S ROOM

1 Where does your baby sleep?
   A In a brand-new crib.
   B On an organic crib mattress.
   C With us.

2 How is the room furnished?
   A From Wal-Mart.
   B With secondhand furniture.
   C With furniture we already had around the home.

3 What DIY materials do you use?
   A Regular paint from the DIY store.
   B Low- or no-VOC paints.
   C Baby-safe eco-paints and bamboo wallpaper.

4 What bodycare products do you use on your baby?
   A Supermarket baby products.
   B Certified organic baby products.
   C Olive oil and Castile soap.

COMMUNITY

1 Who do you socialize with now that you have a baby?
   A We mostly stay at home and stay in touch with people online.
   B We trek across town on the bus to meet up with old friends.
   C We've found many new friends via a local baby-massage group.

2 Where do you hang out?
   A At friends' homes.
   B In a local baby-friendly organic café.
   C At baby reading/play sessions at the local library.

3 Do you use daycare?
   A We travel to a recommended Montessori preschool.
   B We walk to a local playgroup.
   C We set up a local playgroup ourselves.

4 Do you use your local park?

A We use a better one farther away.

B Yes; we've become quite friendly with the local teenagers.

C Yes; we joined a committee to raise money for better facilities.

TRAVEL

1 How do you get to work/school?

A In our car.

B On the bus or train.

C We walk or cycle.

2 Where do you take vacations?

A Wherever we choose.

B At an eco-destination abroad.

C Within this country.

3 What type of fuel does your car use?

A Diesel.

B Biodiesel or electricity.

C What car?

4 How do you get around locally?

A We drive everywhere.

B I have a baby seat on the bike.

C We put the baby in the stroller and walk most places.

ANSWERS

Mostly As

You're not very green yet, but are taking some tentative steps to changing the way you live for the better. Can you change your life a little further now by thinking a little more deeply about some of your lifestyle choices? Try adopting some B and C answers in the future.

Mostly Bs

You're making a good effort at leading a greener life. Perhaps there are a few more simple steps to take you a little farther? Could you cut back on buying brand-new items (even if they are organic), walk more places, and try to reuse things more?

Mostly Cs

You're many times greener than the average family, and so you're making a difference already. Keep up the good work! Who can you pass this book on to once you're finished with it? And what else could you do to become "deep green"? Could you add a layer of sheep's wool insulation to your attic, or even consider generating your own green energy at home?

Caring for your new baby: starting green living from day one

Green health

A greener approach to health means taking a more holistic view of yourself and your baby, and preventing illness before it occurs.

Holistic health involves recognizing that we are part of an ecosystem, and that whatever we put into the environment comes back to us via what we eat, drink, breathe, and absorb through skin; your baby will start to absorb toxins through the placenta while still in the womb. So, caring for the good health of the environment directly benefits us as well. A balanced lifestyle, including a nutritious diet, regular exercise (after your six-week check-up), and a positive attitude, will help keep you and your family happy and in good health.

REST AND RECUPERATION

Aim for two weeks' "lying-in" time to sleep, boost your strength and milk supply by eating healthy meals, and gather your inner resources for the months to come.

It is important to rest adequately after giving birth; this aids recovery, and allows you to bond with your new baby. If you're lucky enough to have a support network, ask for assistance where you need it—most people are only too happy to help. At first, you may want to minimize the number of visitors you have, as they can be extremely tiring. When you do receive guests, you might ask for help with small jobs. Being beholden to others makes it more likely you'll help them in the future, and this forges the close-knit communities that engender green living.

How to ensure good rest

- Set aside a fixed period of postpartum rest, to smooth the transition into motherhood and avoid ill health.
- Climb into a freshly made bed in soft organic cotton pajamas that open down the front for easy breastfeeding.
- Doze when your baby sleeps, rather than trying to get back to your "normal" life.
- Lie skin-to-skin with your baby every day and sing to her; this type of bonding leads to easier breastfeeding and sleeping.
- Spend time gazing into your baby's eyes when she wakes.
- Stop, close your eyes, and allow your breath to become slower and deeper. This relaxed focus will help calm you.
- Ask for a home treatment from a therapist who specializes in postnatal massage, if friends offer to treat you.

Rest is a seriously **undervalued healer** in our super-speedy culture

BABY MASSAGE

Massage is the perfect way to increase confidence in handling tiny limbs, to soothe an unsettled baby, and to promote sleep and development. Choose a time between feedings when your baby is content. You don't need oil for this massage, which is performed over clothes.

1 Sit with your back well supported and knees raised, thighs together. Place your baby tummy-down on your thighs, head turned to one side. Using the back of your right fingers, lightly stroke from your baby's right hip to right shoulder. Follow with your left hand, from left hip to shoulder, and alternate to create a seamless flow of strokes.

2 Taking one foot in your cupped palms, use your thumbs to stroke from toe to heel. Repeat on her other foot.

3 Turn your baby over. With two fingers, trace a square from your baby's right hip to rib cage, across the abdomen, down to the left hip and back to the start. Build up a flowing movement.

4 Take each hand in your palms, and make circles around your baby's palm with your thumbs. Feel them relax as you circle. Talk or sing to her as you work.

Caring for your new baby: Green health

GREEN HEALTH & BODYCARE FOR NEW MOMS

Now that you're a mom, it's important to try to reduce the number of synthetic chemicals you apply to your skin, as these may be transferred to your baby via your milk if you are breastfeeding.

Skin absorbs 60 percent of what's applied to it—80 percent if it's wet. Rub-in (as opposed to rinse-off) products are of particular concern, since it's tricky to find retail cosmetics and bodycare products that don't contain one or more of the following: hormone-disrupting parabens, phthalates toxic to the reproductive system, skin-irritating artificial fragrances, genotoxic formaldehyde, the pesticide triclosan, or various by-products of oil refining. Perhaps surprisingly, many products named "organic" or "natural" still contain synthetic chemicals. To be certain that products are free from these, choose those bodycare items with Soil Association, Demeter, BDIH, Ecocert, or ACO logos.

Replace regular sanitary pads (which contain plastic, bleached wood pulp, pesticide residues, and GM products) with organic disposables, and discard with household waste; flushed pads must be screened out of sewage in municipal treatment plants, and in septic systems, the plastic liner lasts indefinitely.

To reduce landfill waste and manufacturing processes, try washable fair-trade hemp or organic cotton pads (soak in cold water after use, then machine-wash). Once you start having periods again, you might consider a reusable silicone menstrual cup, which functions on a principle similar to a contraceptive cap. For tissues and toilet paper, choose unbleached 100 percent post-consumer recycled; this takes 30–50 percent less energy to produce than paper from trees and cuts pollution into the atmosphere by an incredible 95 percent.

Natural remedies for new moms

In general, there are many natural therapies available (including botanical and homeopathic remedies) that may be helpful for a variety of postpartum conditions. Since each individual responds to certain remedies in different ways, it is always best to consult with your healthcare practitioner on which natural remedy is best for you and your specific ailment. The following conditions may be appropriate for treatment with a natural remedy, but always ask your health care practitioner what he or she would recommend:

- to promote sleep.
- to relieve rough, dry skin.
- to ease shock after giving birth.
- to build up your milk supply.
- to relieve inflamed breasts.
- to ease engorged breasts/mastitis.
- to ease painful or cracked nipples.
- to help with cuts, tears, and bruises.

Caring for your new baby: Green health

GREEN HEALTHCARE FOR BABIES

Increasing numbers of parents are choosing to combine complementary therapies with conventional medicine to treat minor ailments in the first few months of life and throughout childhood.

A kit of healthcare essentials from the herbal and homeopathic pharmocopeia can help tackle the many common childhood illnesses. A typical natural first aid kit might feature items such as aloe vera, calendula, arnica, chamomile, and witch hazel, and all of these products should be available from your local health food store. These items can be useful when in need of first aid for very minor conditions. However, this should in no way be used as a substitute for advice from your healthcare professional. If your baby has a fever, breathing problems, extreme vomiting, or diarrhea, call a doctor at once.

Green medicine cabinets can feature a variety of gentle, natural remedies, which might include botanical or homeopathic treatments. Homeopathic first-aid kits, for example, include

Alternative medicine is popular with parents because it tends to be gentle and have **few side effects**

around 35 remedies for common complaints with a booklet explaining how to use them. These kits can be found at homeopathic pharmacies and health-food stores. Calendula cream and Bach Flower Rescue Remedy can also be valuable additions your green medicine cabinet.

Some parents also use essential oils as part of aromatherapy or infant massage, but do ask your health care practitioner which essentials oils are recommended (and which are contraindicated) for little ones.

Natural remedies for babies

Botanics, homeopathics, and other natural remedies may be effective in helping to ease certain health conditions. It is always essential, however, to consult with your doctor for advice before administering any treatment to your child. The following conditions are a few examples of where a natural remedy may be appropriate for your child, so ask your healthcare practitioner which specific treatment he or she would recommend:

- to relieve nasal congestion.
- to relieve persistent dry, flaky skin.
- to ease colic caused by intestinal gas.
- to help reduce diaper rash.
- to relieve painful teething.
- to promote sleep or ease crying.
- to reduce a fever (when presented with other symptoms).

Caring for your new baby: Green health

Your **natural immunity** can be seriously **compromised** by factors such as **stress**, a high-**sugar** diet, and frequent use of **antibiotics**

IMMUNIZATION

To vaccinate or not to vaccinate may be the first big dilemma you face as a parent. It is interesting that policies vary widely around the world, with certain vaccinations mandatory in some countries but not used at all in others.

Your first step is to become an informed parent by researching the various immunizations using reputable sources and reading the websites of vaccine-awareness groups (see p.185). Do discuss with your doctor concerns you might have regarding links between vaccination and allergies, and the much disputed association with autism. It is important to have an open conversation about the risks and benefits of immunizations. You might ask about how vaccines are produced and what additional ingredients they contain, such as antibiotics, formaldehyde, and mercury. Inquire about common side effects and the latest research on safety, and ask why some parents are so worried that they avoid vaccination or pay for separate shots.

Consider the health of your community, and the risk to other babies and children if you decide not to go ahead with immunization: more than 92 percent of the population must be immune to a virus to prevent an epidemic. If you do choose not to vaccinate, it can be helpful to join a support group of like-minded local parents, who may throw chickenpox or mumps parties to ensure that children catch the diseases in childhood and become immune to them.

Caring for your new baby: Green health

Green baby clothing

Shopping for baby clothes is irresistible, but a young baby doesn't need many items at a time. By buying secondhand, you can keep virgin materials where they belong: on trees and in the ground.

In their first year, babies consume a staggering number of clothes, growing out of garments in three months or less (thankfully, this slows in the second year and beyond). The plus side is that this has given rise to secondhand baby stores, online auctions, and Freecycle sites crammed with beautiful, inexpensive baby clothes, and friends with slightly older babies eager to pass on hardly worn goodies.

For a minimal layette, try four to six bodysuits and sleepers (look for nickel-free poppers), two drawstring sleeping gowns, two to three pairs of pants or dresses, three cardigans, a hat and mittens, and four to six pairs of socks and/or tights. Buy bigger than you think (start with three- to six-month rather than newborn size), and forget shoes until your child starts walking. It's likely you'll be given more stuff than you need. Take some back to exchange for more durable items such as an organic lambskin, or items she will grow into later.

Baby clothes such as hand-knits (see p.39), bamboo shirts (see p.37), and secondhand clothes are all good eco-options.

Caring for your new baby: Green baby clothing

CHOOSING THE GREENEST FIBERS

A brand-new white cotton onesie—what could be purer for a new baby's delicate skin? Well, quite a lot. Unfortunately, brand-new white cotton is far from pure and farther from green.

Cotton doesn't grow well without water, chemical fertilizers, herbicides, defoliants, and pesticides— it uses around 25 percent of the world's insecticides and 11 percent of all pesticides. These pollute the soil, water sources, and marine environment (so also our tap water and the fish we eat), and traces may remain in the finished fabric. Cotton workers (and their babies) are exposed to known carcinogens and developmental toxins. White cotton fabric may be chlorine-bleached, which releases dangerous dioxins into the atmosphere, while colored cotton may contain dyes known to be hazardous to health or skin-sensitizing. And cotton grown in North America, Australia, India, or China may be genetically modified, the risks of which are indeterminate; yet, paradoxically, GM cotton can reduce the impact of pesticides.

One solution is to choose organic cotton. For cotton to be certified organic, it cannot be grown with synthetic chemicals, nor mixed with regular cotton, so it may both feel softer and be of better quality as a result. Look for the Swedish KRAV stamp of approval (Europe's oldest and most prestigious badge of organic production, which guarantees social rights for the producers).

Hemp is the eco-fabric of choice for baby clothes. One of the world's fastest-growing crops (it can be harvested after just 100 days), it produces twice as much fiber per acre as cotton with little need of insecticides, herbicides, or water, and almost all of the plant can be used. A new crop is sown directly after harvesting, for constant renewal of soil carbon, and it leaves the soil weed-free and without excess nitrogen, preventing pollution of water sources. Because hemp fibers are longer than cotton fibers, the fabric is incredibly durable, and clothes tend to keep their shape despite wear and washing. Choose hemp grown in the UK and Europe.

Bamboo fabric feels like silk against precious baby skin and becomes softer with washing, making it ideal for pass-on clothing. Like hemp, it requires minimal pesticides, fertilizers, and water to grow; indeed, it's so hardy that it suits land prone to drought or flooding, and combats soil erosion, helping communities in areas affected by climate change. Bamboo grows quickly (it's harvested every two to five years), takes up little space, and both pumps more oxygen into the atmosphere and traps atmospheric carbon dioxide more effectively than most trees. It absorbs dye easily, reducing the need for chemicals and huge amounts of water. Bear in mind that much of the crop is grown in and transported from East Asia.

Eco clothing solutions

It's not just eco-fabrics that count; being a green parent means thinking about how garments have been made and transported, how durable they are, and the lives of the people who made them.

Be aware of dyes and finishes; if a garment isn't certified organic, it may have been treated with up to 250 heavy metals and synthetic chemicals for easy care, to prevent shrinkage, and to add flame retardance or color. These include hormone disruptors, skin irritants, and carcinogens, which may persist in the environment and pass into our bodies. Avoid any garment with a "new car" smell. Stick to creamy unbleached fabrics in the early days, or those dyed with low-impact vegetable or clay dyes.

"Clothes miles" encompass more than the distance from warehouse to store. Manufacturers—even organic ones—might buy raw materials in one country, then send them across the world for spinning, weaving, or assembly before shipping them back. Favor companies that grow, spin, sew, and sell in one place.

Choose secondhand first. Look for organic cotton or hemp and indulge your label lust sometimes—designer labels create incredibly well-made clothes with smooth seams that pass on better than cheap sweatshop garments. When you buy new, look at a company's ethical trading policy: does it pay a fair price for materials and labor, source locally, and minimize its packaging?

light green Buy new fair-trade unbleached organic cotton garments—the fabric itself contains no traces of harmful chemicals that might irritate your baby's especially sensitive skin, and growing and manufacturing involves very few chemicals. Buying fair-trade also has a positive impact on the farmers who grew the cotton crop (and their families).

 mid green Use secondhand garments passed on from another baby. Look for hemp, a wonder eco-fabric with incredibly durable fibers that keep their shape after washing better than almost any other fabric, giving the garment many potential lives. These garments become softer with wear and are also naturally resistant to harmful UV rays. Remember to pass on to another baby afterward.

deep green Knit your own bootees, hat, or sweater from unbleached pure new wool from a local farm (look for the words "untreated" or "pure grow"). The benefits include canceling out air miles, championing local farmers and heritage breeds, and cutting out garment-manufacture processes—plus, your baby gets a tailor-made garment that you'll want to keep for your next baby or pass on.

Washing baby clothes

For such tiny creatures, babies generate a crazy amount of dirty laundry. To make sure that your laundering is green as well as clean, take care when selecting your washing machine (and dryer, if you need one), and try to adopt sensible laundry habits.

Many parents upgrade their washing machines to coincide with a new baby, but what's the greenest choice now that so many machines have the Energy Star label? Consider the whole life of the machine and its repairability; more expensive manufacturers tend to produce replacement parts that make repairs economical. Budget suppliers may not do this, making machines cheaper to replace than to repair. Also think about where the machine was made. A secondhand machine may be another option, but before you buy, make sure it is energy-efficient.

Line drying baby clothes preserves their life span, and reduces your use of energy-consuming clothes dryers.

Green laundry solutions

The amount of energy we use in washing and drying clothes forms a large (and growing) part of the resources a home consumes—more than 8 percent of electricity and 14 percent of water.

Reducing water temperature is the easiest way to greener laundering, since up to 90 percent of the energy used is to heat the water. Wash most loads at 105°F (40°C), or even 85°F (30°C); use cold water for woolens and delicates, and reserve 140°F (60°C) water for heavily soiled items.

Greener, plant-based detergents, unlike regular petroleum-derived laundry detergents, are made from renewable ingredients that decompose, causing less water pollution. And because they don't contain whiteners, brighteners, or enzymes that attach to clothing, they cause less skin irritation, too. Use half to a quarter of the recommended amount, as a baby's skin is five times thinner than an adult's; if your baby has especially sensitive skin, try none at all. Avoid softener altogether; its skin-irritant ingredients stick to fabric and transfer to baby skin. Laundry-balls and soap nuts are probably the best option, as they require no detergent, softener, or rinse cycle.

Line drying is the greenest way to dry clothes and is also less likely to shrink or damage fibers. Clothes dryers are among the least energy-efficient of all appliances, though laundromat dryers are far better.

light green Put in a full load: each wash uses at least as much water as a bath—around 21 gallons (80 liters) for highly efficient washers, but far more for most machines. Doing fuller loads less often not only saves water and energy, but extends the life span of your washing machine. If you use a dryer, clean the filters as recommended to increase efficiency. Buy electricity from a sustainable source if you can.

mid green Washing a full load at 105°F (40°C) rather than 140°F (60°C) cuts electricity use and carbon emissions by as much as one-third. Use only eco-friendly detergents, and cut back on the amount you use, or try none at all; petroleum-derived fragrances from laundry were detected in 27 percent of streams studied in a US survey. They can irritate delicate new skin and respiratory systems.

 deep green Clothes soiled with baby vomit or worse obviously need washing. But if garments are only lightly soiled, fold them to wear again, and start using bibs. Another plus of washing clothes less often is that they look newer for longer. Real wool and silk garments always need less washing. See if you can reduce your washing machine use from three to four loads a week down to one or two.

Feeding your baby:
the healthiest foods for you, your baby, and the planet

You are what you eat

Humans are at the top of the food chain: grass absorbs nutrients from the soil; a cow eats the grass; we drink its milk. And when your baby drinks your milk, he jumps to the top of the chain.

What's the problem? Put simply, it's that much of our food may be contaminated with low levels of agricultural and industrial chemicals. Some, such as pesticides and growth promoters, may be sprayed onto or injected into crops and livestock; others have leached into the soil through decades of fertilizer and pesticide use, or have been pumped from industrial plants into the atmosphere or rivers, then carried out to sea and absorbed by marine life. Other synthetic chemicals are transferred to food from plastic packaging. Some of the most dangerous chemicals for humans, such as dioxins from chlorine bleaching and PVC manufacturing, persist in the environment indefinitely, since there's nothing to neutralize them.

Many of these environmental toxins seem to get stored remarkably well in the very foodstuffs we need for a healthy diet: oily fish, milk, fruit, and vegetables. After we consume them, the fat-soluble chemicals amass in our bodies over a lifetime—especially in women's bodies, which are naturally fattier than men's— and the only surefire way to detox is if you starve. When you get pregnant or breastfeed, the toxins pass on to your baby.

A 1999 WWF report detected more than 350 synthetic chemicals in breast milk. They included PCBs (found in meat, fish, and dairy food) and alkylphenols (from food packaging) that have the potential to interfere with natural hormone balance, even in very low doses, and may affect the development of the brain and the reproductive and immune systems. Some researchers posit a link with the rise in allergies, autism, behavioral problems, obesity, and early puberty. But no tests have actually been carried out on the safety of multiple exposures to cocktails of industrial chemicals for adults, let alone infants.

Fortunately, there's something positive we can do. First, eat certified organic foods, which are grown without pesticides or many of the synthetic chemicals used to raise conventional crops and livestock. Second, avoid processed foods, which tend to contain artificial additives and be swathed in plastic packaging. Instead, choose fresh, seasonal, local produce; this usually results in reduced carbon emissions, too.

Greenpeace estimates that your **body** may contain up to **200 synthetic chemicals**

EATING ORGANIC

Conventionally farmed fruits and vegetables, both domestic and imported, typically contain residues of multiple pesticides. It's easy to avoid these: just eat organic whenever you can.

Organic farmers are permitted to use only minimal artificial chemical fertilizers and pesticides; animals are reared without nontherapeutic antibiotics or growth hormones; and organic certification guarantees that food is free of genetically modified material. Organic food-processing standards strictly govern what additives can be added to processed foods.

Recent studies suggest that organic foods are higher in nutrients than conventionally farmed produce, with greater amounts of vitamins, minerals, and antioxidants. Researchers found, for example, that organic spinach, cabbage, potatoes, and lettuce have a hugely increased mineral content over conventional crops (up to 100 percent more in spinach), and organic tomatoes have almost double the antioxidant flavonoids. Other studies reported 58 percent more antioxidants in organic fruit, along with double the calcium, four times the magnesium, and 13 times the selenium in organically grown wheat. Organic milk has superstar status, with 68 percent more omega-3 fatty acids than regular milk, plus more vitamins. Pasture-raised organic chicken was found to have 25 percent less fat, and far more flavor.

By nurturing the health of the soil, raising a mixture of crops, and valuing sustainability, organic farming seems to promote good water quality and biodiversity—studies show, for instance, that organic farms shelter more birds, butterflies, and bats than conventional farms. They also provide one-third more local jobs. The organic Rodale Institute even claims that organic farming can significantly reduce emissions of climate-changing gases by conserving more carbon in the soil than regular farming practices, which can deplete carbon content by up to 75 percent.

In a UK poll, more than 70% of consumers reported that organic fruit, vegetables, and meat taste better

Consumer demand is now bringing more organic produce than ever into supermarkets. Look for a "USDA Organic" or "Canada Organic" seal, which guarantees certain environmental and animal-welfare standards. The Demeter Association takes organic principles further, awarding its symbol of biodynamic farming to producers who raise plants to the cycle of the moon, treat soil with homeopathic remedies, and set the needs of workers and community at the center of a holistic vision.

Organic must-haves

- **Dairy foods**—fat-soluble toxins accumulate in fatty foods, so make milk, butter, cheese, and yogurt an organic priority.
- **Meat**—organic meat is free of nontherapeutic antibiotics and growth-promoting hormones, and sausages are made with fewer additives. Stock grazed on pasture, not processed feed, may contain more omega-3 fatty acids (and better flavor).
- **Fruit**—in 2003, all citrus fruit tested in the UK contained pesticide residues, most from multiple sources. Organic fruit isn't waxed or dosed with fungicides after harvesting.
- **Salad leaves**—lettuces are sprayed with more pesticides than any other crop. Washed salads are chlorine-rinsed, and modified-atmosphere packaging can destroy nutrients.
- **Oily fish**—wild salmon and organically farmed salmon and trout contain fewer gender-bending PCBs.
- **Sugary foods**—sugar beets are one of the most heavily-sprayed conventionally farmed crops and provide half the sugar used in the US; sugar-cane production is very polluting and highly damaging to biodiversity.
- **Bread**—organic loaves are free from flour- and dough-improving artificial chemicals and bleaching agents.
- **Whole grains**—conventionally farmed whole grains store a whole dose of pesticides.

Shop locally for organic produce, and take a reusable shopping bag with you.

LABELS AND PACKAGING

Learn how to read and interpret the information on a label, and you can rid your family's diet of many potentially harmful ingredients in food and packaging. Vote with your wallet by boycotting the items below.

Ingredients to avoid

• **Soy**—found in 60 percent of processed foods and in "vegetable" oil, soy may be genetically modified but is not marked as such. Soy is transported around the globe to make feed for intensively reared livestock. Its farming has cleared thousands of square miles of Amazon forest.

• **Sweeteners**—in the US, saccharin is listed as an "anticipated carcinogen"; aspartame can be neurotoxic; high-fructose corn syrup has been linked to diabetes.

• **Trans-fats**—(labelled "partially hydrogenated fats") common in processed foods, these have no nutritional value and are associated with disorders such as coronary heart disease.

• **Synthetic dyes**—a 2007 study linked these food colorings to hyperactivity in children when mixed with the preservative sodium benzoate: FD&C Yellow No. 5, FD&C Yellow No. 6, and to a lesser extent, FD&C Red No. 40.

• **Preservatives**—the following have all been associated with health risks: BHA, BHT, sodium nitrite, sodium nitrate, potassium nitrate, sulfur dioxide, sodium sulfite, sodium metabisulfite, potassium metabisulfite, MSG.

Try to avoid buying food that is packaged—even in biodegradable options, as these only fully degrade when industrially composted (such systems are rare). Plastic packaging, from plastic wrap to plastic bottles and microwavable food trays, is especially harmful to the environment and human health. When PVC (labeled with a "3" in a triangle) is manufactured or destroyed, it pumps dioxins into the atmosphere—exposure can cause human reproductive, developmental, and neurological problems. It also releases heavy metals such as mercury; it is estimated that 1 in 6 newborn babies in the US have levels of mercury high enough to cause brain damage and impair language skills and coordination. The plasticizers (phthalates) that make plastic flexible can be transferred to foods, especially "wet" products (those containing fat). We can inhale them, or they can leach when packaging is heated at high temperatures, and they can scramble normal hormone function. Cans may contain bisphenol-A, an estrogenic chemical that affects the reproductive system in even small doses. Glass and unbleached paper are greener choices.

An Italian study showed that 88% of **newborn babies** tested positive for **plasticizers** in their bodies

Eating local

Eating seasonal local food can be a better option for the health of your baby, your family, and the whole planet than eating organic.

When you eat fresh foods produced locally, you reduce food miles: the distance your dinner travels from all the places it was raised, processed, and packaged to reach your plate. This cuts down on the climate-change emissions caused by transporting food by plane, ship, and truck, and by the refrigeration needed to keep it fresh in transit. It may also decrease the number of postharvest chemicals used to keep produce from spoiling. Fresh ingredients are less likely to be processed or overpackaged, saving the carbon emitted by cooking and chilling, as well as the unrecyclable plastics that usually head straight to a landfill site.

All these factors can make local food greener than organic food. Though more organic produce is now sourced closer to home, the burgeoning popularity of organic food means that much still has to be imported from around the world.

Buying local produce also supports your local community: not only small family farms, but also the specialty shops that stock their products. Without artisan bakers, butchers, and cheesemongers, we would lose a wealth of knowledge about where our food comes from, and how to prepare and cook it.

Supporting local producers also helps to keep their small, local suppliers in business—window cleaners, landscapers, coffee shops—which, in turn, helps preserve a thriving downtown for everyone. If it motivates you, think of buying locally as a form of local fair trade that keeps wealth, services, and even schools in your community.

You're also more likely to be tempted by seasonal food—displays of produce and prices in local stores may vary from month to month, unlike well-stocked supermarkets. Natural therapists extoll the health benefits of eating seasonally; not only do ripe, just-picked fruits and vegetables retain nutrients lost in storage, but because our bodies are adapted to the seasons, we feel better by eating lighter foods in summer and heartier fare in winter.

Why avoid supermarkets? They tend to force down prices paid to suppliers; their demand for perfectly shaped produce renders delicious but homely heirloom apples and carrots worthless; and their centralized distribution increases food miles.

In a German study, it took
5,000 food miles
to bring together the ingredients for
strawberry yogurt

Every $10 you spend in a **local shop** invests $25 in your **community**

But for every $10 spent in a **supermarket** only an extra $4 stays in your **community**

BUYING LOCAL PRODUCE

Buying local produce at bustling farmers' markets, delis, and farm shops makes a very stimulating day out when you have young children.

Support your local farmers' market. Babies in strollers love a lively street market, and it's a great place to meet growers and find out how their crops were cultivated and livestock reared. Plan an afternoon outing to a pick-your-own field or a farm store with refreshments or a petting zoo; look for toddler arts projects linked with seasonal produce, such as pumpkin days in the fall. Visit a specialty deli where staff can tell you which farms your meat came from. Eating less meat is one of the greenest things you can do, since intensive meat production consumes so much water and fossil fuels, and directly causes huge emissions of methane and slurry, a major source of water pollution. Treat meat as a *treat*: take all the money you'd spend on factory-farmed meat at the supermarket and turn it into one high-quality item from a small producer, or try a cheaper cut for slow cooking. While you're out, this is the place to find the ultimate free-range food: rabbit and game.

In the early days of motherhood, home delivery is the best eco-shopping choice: have a local dairy farm deliver milk in returnable, toxin-free glass bottles, and subscribe to a weekly CSA produce box. You could even set yourself a challenge to see if you can source everything you eat from within 100 miles.

Feeding your baby: Eating local

Growing your own

The most local food is the food you grow in your own backyard—and you don't need acres to do this. A few pots and window boxes can yield a surprisingly large amount of produce, from potatoes to exotic berries.

More and more families are eager to trace their food from soil to fork: increasing numbers of mail-order companies offer heirloom fruit and vegetable seeds, and more community gardens are offering city-dwellers the chance to grow their own produce. You might quake at the thought of giving yourself any extra work, but growing in pots is relatively hassle-free (no digging and little weeding). And if you buy young plants, you cut out the worry about whether seeds will germinate (though toddlers love that part). Involve your baby in planting and watering; let her get muddy. If you can't deal with soil, sprout seeds in a jar—toddlers relish the juicy crunch of sprouted garbanzos.

Easy crops children love to grow
• Tumbling cherry tomatoes in hanging baskets.
• Potatoes or garlic in half-barrels, or carrots in large pots (an effective natural barrier to carrot root fly).
• Lettuces and green onions in a window box.

As well as learning about the seasons and how food grows, children exposed to soil may be less prone to allergies.

- Blueberry bushes in pots of ericaceous soil, or soil-planted apple trees native to your region.
- Basil raised from seed on a window sill.
- Alfalfa sprouts in a sprouting vessel such as a jar.

Cooking at home

Home-cooking is the greenest habit we can cultivate, as cooking from scratch allows us to choose the best ingredients, ditch unnecessary packaging, and pass on invaluable skills.

The essence of good home-cooking is really great ingredients: butter instead of low-fat spread; fresh eggs, not egg substitute. When ingredients are fresh, ripe, and pure (meaning local, in season, and unprocessed), they are full of natural flavor and need only minimal cooking—saving fuel and retaining maximum nutrients. Sales of packaged convenience foods continue to rise, yet with a tasty loaf of bread, some ripe home-grown tomatoes, and a chunk of regional cheese, you have lunch. Add a salad, a home-made soup, and a plate of seasonal berries with local yogurt; now you have a feast.

This type of cooking involves knowing what's best when: When is asparagus in season? When can you pick blackberries? It's also about cultivating the art of conjuring up delicious dishes from leftovers. One study found that the average household throws away about 1¼ lb (550 g) of food every day; most of this goes into a landfill. Finally, don't leave the microwave plugged in: it uses more energy for the clock than in cooking.

Engage your toddler when preparing food, so she learns the pleasures of home-cooking early.

Eco shopping solutions

Food and drink production is thought to be responsible for about one-third of a family's overall environmental impact. The fair-trade movement says we can change the world by shopping selectively; use the power of your purse to start reducing the impact your family makes.

To avoid endangered fish species, check one of the online guides to buying eco-friendly seafood from sustainable sources (see p.186). Also try to avoid long-line and trawler-caught pelagic fish—trawling in particular causes the death of dolphins, turtles, and other marine mammals. Fish that is line-caught by hand is the best choice.

The way people in your region have eaten for centuries has molded the landscape: the livestock raised and crops grown determine the look of fields and fencerows. To preserve the countryside, buy traditional foods that support small farms. If we don't, farms may turn into subdivisions, fields become golf courses or parking lots, and communities start to falter.

To change the world farther afield, try some fair-trade fruit, sugar, coffee, tea, and cocoa. Fair-trade companies bring ethically raised food to a world market, helping to bring employment and prosperity to farmers and their regions. Fair terms are agreed for products, and environmental standards are often good.

light green Buy organic foods from a supermarket, choosing locally grown produce over imported goods. Reject items flown in from overseas (air freighting has a much greater environmental impact than transportation by sea or road). Select food with little or no packaging, and check that what packaging there is can be completely recycled (or leave it behind at the checkout).

mid green Shop at your local farmers' market to cut your number of trips to suburban supermarkets and support your community's agricultural economy. At the grocery store, again, favor locally produced goods (food miles rose by 15 percent between 1992 and 2002) and foods with less packaging. Always take along a fabric bag or basket to bring your groceries home.

 deep green Grow some of your own food, gather wild foods if possible, and swap with friends. Supplement with a CSA subscription from a nearby farm. A vegetarian meal cooked from all-local ingredients has top eco-credentials, a 2003 Swedish study found, equating to around just 6½ oz (190 g) carbon dioxide release; a meaty meal made of mostly imported ingredients increased the carbon load to 4 lb (18 kg).

Breastfeeding

Breastfeeding couldn't be more environmentally beneficial; it means no food miles, no packaging, no need for washing or detergents, no reliance on formula made by multinational conglomerates, no electricity-guzzling refrigerator or sterilizer— for six whole months or more.

What's not to like? Well, it can hurt at first, be hard to master without expert help, and confine you to hours on the sofa and wakeful nights. Breastfed babies tend to wake more often through the night, feed more frequently during the day, and can take less readily to scheduled feedings than bottle-fed babies.

But consider the superlative health benefits for mother and baby. Breast milk provides the perfect mix of nutrients, as well as protection against infections and environmental contaminants. From the first feeding onward, breastfed babies benefit. They tend to be more intelligent, healthier, and more resistant to infections, allergies, diabetes, and obesity. Even if only breastfed for one month, their health is improved up to age 14, compared with babies who have not been breastfed at all.

Breastfeeding deepens the bond between mother and baby as well as providing long-term health benefits for both.

Feeding your baby: Breastfeeding

Breastfeeding mothers also reduce their own risk of osteoporosis and cancer of the breast and ovaries, and get back in shape more quickly after the birth. Most mothers who give up breastfeeding say they would have liked to have kept it up for longer, but lacked support. The best help comes in person; day or night, call your hospital's breastfeeding counselor. If you're out of the hospital, call a breastfeeding helpline (see p.186)—these are staffed by trained, experienced breastfeeding mothers. Or you might drop in on a breastfeeding coffee morning, where other mothers can reassure you. Alongside the confidence that comes with expert advice, the key to success in breastfeeding consists of perseverance, patience, and willpower.

It's helpful to know that your baby's "weird" feeding habits are completely normal

There are considerable advantages to breastfeeding beyond weaning. Even when solid food is providing your baby's main nourishment, breast milk continues to confer immunity from germs (in studies, breastfed toddlers get ill less often than other children). It is also a lovely way for your child to feel nurtured when she's venturing out into the world. If your only feedings are before bed and first thing in the morning, each day begins and ends in a loving, green way, and you may even be able to bypass bottles altogether.

EXPRESSING MILK

Want to breastfeed and still have a life? Try expressing some milk. This way, dads also get a chance to nurture their baby with nature's most renewable resource.

Allow a few weeks to establish breastfeeding before you attempt expressing milk. To find out how to express by hand (the greenest way), ask a breastfeeding expert or look online (see p.186). However, many mothers prefer to use a handheld pump, which gently draws the milk into an attached bottle. Another reason to express is to build your milk supply: pump after feeding, and in a few days you'll make enough milk for your baby, plus extra to freeze. Expressing also relieves aching breasts of overabundant milk. But don't feel discouraged if you can't express—some of us just can't—or if your baby refuses a bottle; he may accept it from someone else.

Breastfeeding kit

- **Nursing bra**—buy at least two (get them fitted by a professional) and try out the organic options.
- **Breast pads**—washable silk, wool, bamboo, or hemp feel softer against delicate skin than paper disposables.
- **Expressing machines**—borrow first to see which you prefer: speedy hospital-style pumps or hand pumps.
- **Storage jars**—use lidded glass bottles; more immunity properties are preserved by refrigerating than by freezing.

Feeding your baby: Breastfeeding

SUPERFOODS FOR BREASTFEEDING

Superfoods are those that are considered especially
nutritious or beneficial to health. By eating the right foods
when breastfeeding, you can stay in shape, build a
healthy supply of milk, and protect the planet, too.

You need around 300–400 extra calories a day for the first
three months of exclusive breastfeeding. To be sure you are
eating a balanced diet, these calories should come from a
variety of foodstuffs; if you select local and seasonal produce,
which varies your diet as different items come into season,
you will effortlessly achieve a good mix of nutrients.

Left to right: calcium-rich yogurt also contains healthy bacteria; lemons (unwaxed)
provide vitamins C and A; Swiss chard is high in vitamins and minerals; red
peppers contain antioxidants; oily fish boasts essential omega-3 fatty acids; and oats
are a good source of soluble fiber as well as a range of vitamins.

Essential foods

- **Fruit and vegetables**—aim for more than five a day, including some green leafy vegetables and orange, red, or yellow produce. Organic means far fewer pesticide residues, and since fruit and vegetables are the largest category of air-freighted goods, try to choose local produce, too. However, do note that it can be greener to import foods that grow easily in warmer regions (e.g., tomatoes, citrus fruit) than to grow them in far northern climates in heated greenhouses.
- **Oily fish**—eat about twice a week, choosing from a variety of smaller fish that harbor fewer toxins, such as sardines, herring, and anchovies.
- **Whole grains**—seek out organic loaves with no soy flour, enjoy organic oats for breakfast, and try grains like spelt.
- **Dairy produce**—organic is free from hormones; natural yogurt has more calcium than milk.

Eating **conventionally farmed** foods means that your **breast milk** could contain **higher levels of dioxins** than those permitted in pasteurized **cow's milk**

AVOIDING TOXINS

The idea of banned toxins in breast milk is frightening. Do you need to worry? And what can you do to green your life and detox your chemical load?

All breast milk contains measurable levels of industrial chemical contaminants, wherever you live and whatever your lifestyle. This is because fat stores toxins very well, making naturally fatty breast milk an important indicator of the levels of contaminants in our food chain. These contaminants leach out of paints and industrial detergents, from pesticides and PVC plastic, and seep into our bodies via our skin and through the stuff we eat from high up in the food chain. So the toxins in breast milk merely reflect the general level of environmental pollution. This does not mean that you should stop breastfeeding, which boosts immunity and thus helps limit damage from environmental pollutants. What you *can* do is campaign for more research into the effects of synthetic toxins. Join the WWF, write to your representative, or start a blog. We can only clean up the environment by getting together and acting globally. Take some practical measures to minimize your direct toxin intake, too. Eat organic foods and use safe bodycare products (see p.28); spend less time close to electronic equipment and plastic; avoid large oily fish with mercury residue (stick to smaller fish such as sardines); and decorate with eco-paints. Above all, stop smoking and make your home a smoke-free zone.

Feeding your baby: Breastfeeding

Holistic bottle-feeding

An advantage of bottle-feeding is that dads, grandparents, and other caregivers can also bond with your baby, whether using expressed breast milk or formula milk.

There are various reasons why some women are unable to breastfeed; and even those who can may decide it is just not practical all the time. The easiest way to make bottle-feeding a more personal experience is by ensuring some skin-to-skin contact as you nestle together, to promote intimacy and stimulate your baby's sense of smell and touch.

The synthetic toxins found in breast milk have been well publicized, but that is not to say that formula milks have any less of a toxic load. In fact, since most formula is made from cow's milk, it will be prone to the same type of contaminants. You may add more into the mix from tap water, formula containers, and the actual bottle, even if the ingredients of the powder are all organic. The cultivation, processing, and packaging of formula milk may also shed carbon dioxide and toxins into the environment; fossil fuels are burned in manufacture, transportation, and refrigeration, forests are cleared for cattle-grazing, and packaging is bleached and printed on.

Very few babies are born with lactose intolerance, but even if your baby is, try to avoid soy-based formula. Intensive

Always make up a fresh bottle of formula milk for each feeding, and consider using a water filter for tap water.

cultivation of the crop in Brazil has resulted in the destruction of pristine rainforest and widespread rural unemployment. Soy accounts for the highest percentage of pesticide sales worldwide, and much of the crop is genetically modified (even when not labeled as such); no trials have been done on the safety of GM material for infants. Soy milk also contains plant estrogens, which certain studies have shown can affect the development of a baby's reproductive system and the brain. Goat's-milk formula is no longer recommended as an alternative, as it still contains some lactose. Speak to your healthcare provider about selecting an appropriate formula for your baby.

For the bottle itself, strengthened glass bottles are the greenest choice (see p.186). Most baby bottles (95 percent) are made from polycarbonate plastic (marked with a "7" in a triangle). This contains bisphenol-A, an estrogen-mimicking chemical that can have adverse effects on development at even very low doses; it may leach into milk when the bottles are heated or scratched. A better plastic is polypropylene (marked with a "5"). It's one of the plastics with the lowest impact on the environment, and it doesn't contain any bisphenol-A.

By 4–10 weeks, **75%** of mothers either use infant formula entirely or combine it with breastfeeding

STERILIZING

All bottle-feeding equipment should be sterilized for your baby's first year, as milk can get encrusted in the grooves and become a breeding ground for bacteria. However, when you start weaning your baby (at six months or older), you won't need to sterilize his bowls and spoons.

Look for bottles you can put directly into the microwave, the most energy-efficient form of heating, and use a microwave steam sterilizer. (Don't use the microwave to heat a bottle of milk or formula, though—hidden hot spots in the liquid could burn your baby's mouth.) To sterilize without buying any new equipment, set aside a large pan and boil items in it for ten minutes (though this destroys nipples very quickly). Using the dishwasher is not the greenest option: it has to run at 175°F (80°C) to sterilize. Solar kettles have been an important advancement for sterilizing water in developing countries.

Immunity-boosting tips

• Breastfeed for as long as possible, if you are able.
• Sterilize bottles but don't be too neurotic about cleanliness; your baby needs exposure to germs to develop immunity.
• Avoid antibiotics unless absolutely necessary.
• Consult a homeopath about treatments that will strengthen your baby's constitution.

Feeding your baby: Holistic bottle-feeding

Green weaning

Babies need nothing other than milk for the first six months of life. Then things get interesting (but more messy) as you introduce them to the world of good eco-food.

You'll know when your baby is ready for something more than milk by the way she watches you eating and mimics chewing or reaches out for food. Don't be tempted to start your baby on solid food before the age of six months (talk to your healthcare provider if you have concerns or if your baby was born prematurely): babies weaned after six months are less likely to develop food allergies.

Try to make your baby's first tastes organic. Researchers from the University of Washington found that children who ate organic food had six times less pesticide residue in their bodies than those fed on nonorganic foods. The standards for tolerable levels of pesticides on foods are based on what's considered safe for adults. No research has been done to determine safety for infants, nor any tests into the effects of long-term exposure to low-level cocktails of chemicals. Babies may be more at risk, not just because the brain and immune system are vulnerable during development, but because babies eat more in proportion to their size, and an immature digestive system absorbs toxins effectively but undeveloped organs aren't able to eliminate them very readily.

The Environmental Working Group states that the greatest pesticide risk comes from just 12 foods

The traditional way to start weaning is to offer a little baby rice cereal mixed to a sloppy consistency with your baby's regular milk. Don't force it: babies get all the nutrients they need from milk up to the age of one. When your baby is happily eating baby rice cereal, you can gradually add pureed fruit and vegetables and other grains one by one, waiting a few days to check for reactions before adding a new food. After eight months, try protein-rich food, such as organic chicken, lentils, eggs, cheese, and yogurt.

That said, many parents are now choosing to ignore the guidance on purees (developed when we started weaning at three or four months, when babies can't hold up their heads or manipulate well from hand to mouth). Instead, they offer finger foods: bite-sized chunks of food that the baby feeds herself. This is known as baby-led weaning. Whichever approach you choose, offer cooked vegetables (especially) and fruit before you start your baby on proteins, and make sure to buy organic when it comes to the pesticide "dirty dozen": peaches, apples, bell peppers, celery, nectarines, strawberries, cherries, lettuce, grapes, pears, spinach, and potatoes.

Feeding your baby: Green weaning

SUPERGREEN FINGER FOODS

Babies weaned directly onto finger foods are less likely to be fussy eaters, say advocates of this method, because they learn to cope with the texture and taste of real food from the outset.

Giving your baby finger foods is certainly less stressful than lovingly preparing a puree, only to watch it being spat out and smeared over the table. Start by offering your baby foods cut into french-fry shapes for easy grasping. You could try steamed broccoli or carrot, roast squash, or a hunk of "real" bread (not supermarket bread made by the industrial method, which lacks flavor and texture), perhaps smeared with some hummus or avocado. Make sure you always sit at the table as your baby gums and sucks the food in case he gags (a safety reflex to prevent choking). The reason baby-led weaning seems to be so effective is that your baby eats alongside you—and the same food as you—from day one, rather than getting fixated on sweet, bland purees. Your baby also takes control, choosing what to eat and how much, which means you lose some control. This method of weaning is much messier than offering neat spoonfuls of puree, and wiping the mouth after each one, but have courage!

Start your baby on finger foods, and he's more likely to become an adventurous eater.

Feeding your baby: Green weaning

MAKING FIRST PUREES

When you make your own baby food from fresh fruit or vegetables, you can reassure yourself about their provenance: for this method, you could use apples, carrots, squash, or other produce. Use a hand-powered mill, which requires no electricity and allows you to vary the texture for your growing baby.

1 Wash the produce very well, scrubbing with a brush reserved for this task. Peel all nonorganic orchard fruit and root vegetables. Remove seeds or pits, or core fruit.

2 Steam the vegetables or fruit for a few minutes until quite soft but not falling apart. Or you could simmer in a scant amount of water instead.

3 Grind the vegetables or fruit with the hand-powered mill until you have a puree with a consistency appropriate for your baby's age.

4 Spoon enough for one meal into your baby's bowl, adding milk or cooking water if necessary. Store the remainder in the refrigerator in clean, lidded glass jars for up to two days, or freeze immediately in a non-plastic ice-cube tray (label with the date and use within six months).

Feeding your baby: Green weaning

Eco baby food solutions

Baby food is now the single largest sector of the organic market, and growing numbers of the jars of baby food on the shelves have been certified organic, which is very reassuring. But which are the greenest options for feeding your baby?

Not all organic baby food is the same. Before you buy, make sure to read the label, checking the ingredients list and the expiration date. There's a world of difference between jars of food that were processed from cheap and bulky root vegetables and lots of water before you even got pregnant, and freshly made food with quality ingredients with real flavor. In this case, the ultimate test of quality is the taste test. Buy a few different jars and have them for lunch. If you wouldn't eat the food yourself, why give it to your baby, who has many times the number of taste buds you have? If you can afford it, always choose baby foods with the shortest shelf life (some stay fresh for just days). However, if you have the option, cooking your baby's food yourself is the greenest and tastiest course of action, whether you opt for purees and reusable storage jars or think outside the jar and head straight to finger foods. Cooking with seasonal ingredients not only helps the environment, but also ensures that your baby meets an ever-changing variety of foods, lessening the risk of overexposure to pesticide residues from any single ingredient.

light green Buy jars of organic food from the supermarket. The greenest choices probably won't have been heat-processed, and so you're more likely to find them in the chiller case or freezer; these are most likely to taste like "real" food. Or, better yet, if you shop at a nearby farm or organic supermarket, you might even come across a range made locally.

 mid green Make your own baby food from local, seasonal organic ingredients. This saves food miles and the fossil fuels spent in industrial production processes. Feeding your baby seasonal foods has health benefits, too: Austrian research shows that produce picked in season is higher in nutrients (especially vitamin C, which degrades in transit) than flown-in ingredients.

deep green Ditch special baby foods and give your child the home-cooked food you eat (with less salt), dining together as a family as often as you can. Change your recipes with the seasons or according to what arrives in your weekly CSA box. Show your baby how good home-cooked dishes taste (whether organic or not) and you are setting him up to eat well for life.

Eating as a family

Before your baby celebrates his first birthday, you have a window of opportunity to influence his eating habits for life. Will he prefer processed tastes or be prepared to try anything?

If everyone in your household sits at a table together, your baby will recognize the sociable, bonding properties of eating long before he smears his first fistful over his face. Even if you can't eat as a family all the time, you can still turn off the TV (a great green habit); sit at a table; set the table with cutlery (with utensils for your baby too); not have anything else on the table (no books or toys); and decide when the meal ends. It may be easier to allow finger foods in front of the TV, but it's a habit your child may still be in by his early teens. Cut out processed food, and above all, eat together and eat the same food so you don't lead two food lives—now that's green!

Making mealtimes calm occasions when you share time as well as food leads to more adventurous eaters and less food in the trash.

GREEN MEALTIME EQUIPMENT

Mealtimes with a baby at the table mean a little more equipment is required. Here are the green items to prioritize, from high chairs to sippy cups.

Bibs are essential if you're not to add to your laundry load. There are fair-trade organic cotton versions, or try tying an old-fashioned adult apron around your baby's neck (to cover him to his toes); pick them up at secondhand stores. Some babies like a hard pelican-style bib they can retrieve fallen food from (hard plastic contains fewer plasticizing chemicals than flexible plastic).

Plastic bowls are never good for the environment—their manufacture and incineration sheds toxins into the environment that endanger human health. Some campaigners worry that plasticizing chemicals in plastic baby bowls might leach into food, especially when a bowl is scratched. Don't heat food in plastic, either: decant it into a heat-proof container instead. You might like to try a fair-trade bamboo baby bowl and cutlery set or a stainless steel bowl, which will last forever. As your baby gets older, he might even graduate to ceramic bowls (in the plural; don't get too attached to them, as there are likely to be breakages). If you're worried about potential toxins in plastic sippy cups, choose one made from plastic other than polycarbonate plastic (avoid those marked with a "7" in a triangle). Or, you can search online for stainless steel versions (which also don't taint the drink with a plastic taste, and are reassuringly resilient).

You might not need a high chair when you start giving your baby her first taste of solid food—he'll be happy to sit on your lap to begin with—but as soon as he can sit unsupported, he'll enjoy having his own space at the table (even if the food doesn't stay there). The world's best-selling children's chair, the wooden Stokke Trip Trap, is the greenest because it "grows" with your baby; you can adjust it to bring him to the perfect level for eating at an adult table as a baby, toddler, preschooler, schoolchild, and even as a teenager or adult. And it's a design classic that will still look good at a table when your children have left home. Baby chairs that clip to the side of the table use fewer raw materials than a full-size chair, are portable, and also ensure that your baby eats at a table like you, not at a plastic tray (though prepare for a mess on the table and food sliding around). Avoid chairs with vinyl, padding, and frills that just get food-infested (chairs you can shoot a shower-jet at are best for ease of cleaning).

It's handy to put something under the high chair to catch at least some of the mess. If you don't want plastic in your green home, use recyclable newspaper or find a square of linoleum (which is quite eco-friendly, as it's made with linseed oil and jute, and is completely biodegradable).

The green, clean baby: gentler approaches to washing and cleaning

What is clean?

US studies suggest that the air inside homes can be many times more polluted than outdoor air, even in cities. This has much to do with the chemical cocktail of cleaning products we use.

80% of most people's exposure to pesticides occurs when they are indoors

Most cleaning products available in supermarkets are chock-full of ingredients that aren't good for the environment or your baby. Most non-eco cleaners contain petroleum-derived surfactants (detergents), such as SLS, that don't readily biodegrade or may form dangerous compounds as they do so. They may also contain hormone-disrupting phthalates, phosphates, musks, or colorings (none of which has to be detailed on the label). The effects of polluted indoor air are worst for those who spend most of their time indoors, and the very young. Living in an over-clean home in the first year of life is also associated with a heightened risk of allergies and asthma. Epidemiologists say that our high standards of cleanliness (and small family size) mean that babies are less exposed to germs now than in the past, with the result that their underused immune systems may then over-respond to common substances such as pollen and dust. Chemicals in cleaning products have also been linked to asthma. Don't throw the iffy ones in the trash (straight into a landfill) or down the drain (into the water supply); see if your waste collection service accepts hazardous chemicals, or call a local environmental awareness group for advice (see p.185).

What to toss out

- **Cleaning fluids**—(even eco ones) containing glycol ethers, terpenes, or limonenes (in pine or citrus scents); a 2006 report said they create toxic air conditions in confined space.
- **Air fresheners**—young babies exposed to air fresheners have been found to be prone to diarrhea and ear infections.
- **Chlorinated ingredients**—look for the term "chlor-" in heavy-duty products such as bleaches. The manufacturing process is deadly and chlorine reacts with organic material to create compounds hazardous to the environment.
- **Anti-pest products**—whether for home, garden, or pets, they are likely to contain pesticides (-*cide* means "killer").
- **Antimicrobials**—don't clean better than soap and water, and are banned in some hospitals because it is feared they lead to superbugs. They can contain up to 275 pesticides, and traces have been found in breast milk and fish.
- **Aerosols**—blast neuro- and reproductive toxins and respiratory irritants directly into the respiratory tract.

Greener home cleaning

There are many effective green cleaning products you can buy—but you might find the most eco-friendly already on your own kitchen shelves.

When there's a baby in the house, shop for green cleaning products that suit people sensitive to dyes and fragrances. Buy products at a place where you can refill them, or choose concentrates in smaller bottles, since the largest component in household cleaners is water—that's a lot of carbon dioxide expended on transporting colored water. You might like to inquire about the manufacturer's animal-testing policy (some claim that to make products greener, they have to use newer ingredients that need to be animal-tested).

Be aware of the air in a room when you're cleaning, especially if your baby is with you: his respiratory system is immature, and humidity increases the chances of irritant ingredients penetrating his respiratory tract. Avoid products that spray into the air; be sure to rinse very well; and open windows, especially if your home is green and well insulated, keeping them open for a few hours, until the smell disappears. Store used cleaning cloths well out of the way of inquisitive hands. Also pay attention to the floor—the place where babies spend a large part of their first couple of years, when their brain, internal organs, and immune system are developing. Any products sprayed indoors eventually settle on the floor, as do toxins tracked in from outdoors on shoes. These then mingle with dust from computers and other electronic equipment that may be laced with flame-retardant chemicals linked to reproductive and neurological disorders.

Consider ridding your home of carpets. The largest dust reservoir in a home, a typical carpet contains high levels of heavy metals such as lead, pesticides, PCBs (linked with impaired cognitive abilities in infants), and PAHs (from car exhaust and smoking, associated with DNA damage).

Children playing or crawling on carpets may ingest 5 times more dust than adults

If your carpets are providing important insulation to your home, just bear in mind that 25 strokes with a powerful vacuum cleaner are needed every week for a few weeks to detox a carpet. One of the easiest ways to reduce the toxins and dirt entering your home is to instigate a shoes-off policy. Buy a deep doormat and leave indoor shoes or slippers by the door.

Green cleaners

- **White vinegar**—dilute with water to make a wipe for surfaces, glass, and tiles, or use full-strength to unclog showers and sinks. The smell disappears as it evaporates.
- **Lemon juice**—squeeze onto surfaces and cutting boards to degrease and for a bleaching effect.
- **Salt**—use for washing dishes or to scour baked-on food.
- **Spices**—simmer a handful of dry spices (try cinnamon sticks, cloves, fresh ginger root, cardamom seeds, star anise), or slices of lemon, lime, and orange to scent your home.
- **Bicarbonate of soda**—mix into a paste for sinks and tubs, or sprinkle into the toilet bowl, add white vinegar, and scrub.
- **Microfiber miracle cloths**—just dampen and rub. These need no solvents or detergents to get rid of grease and stubborn stains. Wash in the washing machine when dirty.
- **Wet-dusting solution**—mop with liquid Castile soap, then rinse with water plus 10 drops essential oil of grapefruit.
- **Raise a plant**—many broad-leaved house plants neutralize airborne toxins like formaldehyde and benzene.
- **Shake and vac**—sprinkle bicarbonate of soda over carpet, leave for a couple of hours, then vacuum.
- **Toilet-seat spray**—add 10 drops of antibacterial tea tree essential oil to water in a mister, shake, then spritz.

Encourage your young child to help with the household chores so that she feels she is a valued member of the family cleaning team.

Washing your baby

Babies don't need a bath every day until they start crawling (when they can get filthy quickly). In the early days, save water and protect your baby's skin by simply topping and tailing daily.

Topping and tailing is an easy and eco-friendly way to keep your baby clean (see pp.98–99), and cuts down on the number of baths your baby needs until she starts getting really dirty with the onset of solid food and crawling. At least until this point, no baby needs commercial cleansing products: yes, that really does mean no soap, baby bubbles, shampoo, lotions, or oils. Many cleansers— or even too much tap water—can irritate or damage a baby's delicate skin. The barrier layer of skin is immature during the first year of life and absorbs water more readily than mature skin, making it vulnerable to irritants and water-soluble toxins in skincare products. It also loses moisture more quickly, so the fewer drying detergents, the better. Plain warm water is usually enough to get rid of most messes, and organic olive oil makes a good wipe for stuck-on stuff and is emollient for dry skin. As a

An infant's skin does not develop a barrier to environmental toxins for 2–3 years last resort, use a small amount of organic baby soap. Some parents like to use natural sponges, which are gentle on the skin, biodegradable, and compostable.

A slippery baby and unconfident parent make a scary combination, while plastic baby baths can be cold and hard for a baby (as well as nonsustainable). Many green parents find sharing a bath with their baby is a more bonding, friendly, and secure experience (it saves water, too). Bathing together can soothe an agitated baby and help lift parental exhaustion in the evening. Keep the water tepid (around 100°F/ 38°C) and don't add any oils or bubbles. Turning down the thermostat on your water heater to 120°F (49°C) earns you extra eco-points.

Get into the tub, then have someone pass you the baby. Cuddle your baby in the water at first, keeping her body and shoulders submerged, but resting on you until you both feel more relaxed. Then swim her through the water, with her head and neck firmly supported. When your baby is able to sit up, sit her opposite you in waist-high water and sink down so that your faces are at the same level; this makes a great opportunity to talk to each other. Ask your baby a question and see how she answers with splashes. When you're done bathing, pass your child to an adult waiting with a warmed hooded towel to dry and dress her in warmed clothes while you climb out. Babies lose body heat very quickly. Never leave your baby or toddler unattended in or near a bathtub, or even turn your back on her for a moment.

TOPPING AND TAILING

Cleaning your baby's face, hands, and bottom is all that's needed in the early weeks and protects her new skin from harsh detergents. You'll need two soft, clean washcloths, a warmed towel, some fair-trade cotton balls, a little organic olive oil, and a warm room.

1 Undress your baby to the waist. Wipe her face and around her neck creases carefully with a damp, warm washcloth. Dry with a warmed towel. Wipe each eye very gently from the center outward with separate moistened cotton balls. Repeat on her nostrils, if necessary.

2 If your baby's hair needs freshening up, dampen the washcloth and wipe from the front of her head to the nape of her neck. Pat dry with a warm towel.

3 Wipe your baby's hands and under her arms with the washcloth. Carefully pat dry. If your baby has areas of dry skin, rub on some organic olive oil. Clothe her upper body.

4 Undress your baby from the waist down. Moisten another flannel and wipe her bottom from front to back. Pat dry with the towel, then rub a little of the olive oil on any areas of diaper rash. Put her in a clean diaper and dress her.

Eco baby wipe solutions

Baby wipes are one of the most wasteful products on the planet—after all, they are designed to be thrown away. Studies show that it's best not to use them for at least the first month of life. Here are some greener options.

Conventional baby wipes made of bonded plastic, cellulose, and polyester don't biodegrade: each one can take several hundred years to break down, and the average baby uses up to 5,000 in her lifetime. Most conventional brands also tend to be chlorine-bleached: industrial bleaching has seriously damaged the environment and caused the release of POPs (persistent organic pollutants) that remain indefinitely in our soil, water, food, and bodies, and are linked with learning and behavioral problems.

When parents were interviewed for a 2007 report on chemicals in baby products, almost 90 percent said that they read the ingredients labels on food, but only a third regularly inspected skincare products. Nearly half severely underestimated the number of synthetic chemicals in even "gentle" baby wipes—there may be more than 15. These include the skin-irritating SLS (sodium lauryl sulfate), synthetic fragrances, propylene glycol (which enhances the penetration of other chemicals into the skin), estrogen-mimicking parabens, and pesticide-heavy antibacterial agents.

light green Choose eco-brands that are unbleached, completely biodegradable and flushable, made with purified water and cleansing agents derived from sugar and vegetable oils, and with organic skin-soothing botanicals, such as aloe vera. Use them mainly for trips out rather than home use. Buying refill packs means 90 percent less packaging.

mid green Make your own wipes from one of the many online recipes, using unbleached, recycled paper towels, cider vinegar, calendula oil, and aloe vera. Store in an old plastic wipe box. Alternatively, buy a diluted sea-water spray, spritz onto an organic cotton cloth, and use to wipe her bottom or hands. Or make your own wipe-spray (see pp.106–107) and store in the refrigerator in a reusable glass bottle.

deep green Gently clean your baby's bottom with recycled toilet paper, dispose of it in the toilet, then wipe with a washable organic flannel cloth moistened with plain water (throw it in the diaper pail). For sticky hands and faces, moisten another clean, organic cloth (if you're going out, it's easily transported in a waterproof bag).

Every single week, a baby will get through, on average, 42

disposable diapers

In the US alone, around

50 million disposables are

dumped in landfills

each day

Greener diapers

Change your baby into reusable diapers, and you can change the world at the same time by greatly reducing landfill waste and carbon emissions.

Most of the waste a baby generates derives from disposable diapers, which make up a significant portion of a family's garbage. This enormous amount of waste can take 200–500 years to decompose—imagine all the untreated sewage and harmful methane produced by the billions of diapers in landfills (diapers are the third-largest global contributor to landfill sites). The energy and resources consumed in the manufacture of disposable diapers are also considerable, since they are made largely from polypropylene plastic and bleached, pulped wood. The chemical load of conventional disposable diapers often includes superabsorbent granules of sodium polyacrylate (banned from tampons for health reasons), bactericides, pesticides, and deodorants associated with skin irritation and allergic reactions.

Despite claims to the contrary (mainly from disposable diaper companies), reusable diapers are kinder by far to the environment, and to your baby's skin. Real diapers can reduce your climate-change impact by a quarter. And you're likely to need diapers for fewer months, too: babies who wear washables tend to potty-train earlier (because they learn what it's like to feel wet from an early age).

The green, clean baby: Greener diapers

CHOOSING A DIAPER

So which washables will you choose? Organic cotton, bamboo, and hemp are sound eco-options. As well as being the world's most green crops (see p.37), bamboo and hemp are naturally antibacterial and hypoallergenic. Bamboo absorbs 60 percent more moisture than cotton and does it more quickly than cotton (the diapers dry twice as fast, too), while hemp improves in absorbency and softness with washing. Silk diaper liners wick away moisture from skin better than other fabrics; and soft woolen outer wraps offer natural water-resistance, breathability, and antibacterial properties, and often can be aired rather than washed.

Washable diapers are the cheapest green-diaper option in the long run (though the initial investment may seem higher) and you'll save even more if you use them on subsequent babies. Secondhand cloth diapers can be found for sale online. Most modern washable diapers are shaped like disposables, with easy fasteners and no need for expertise in origami, and there are sizes to suit every infant, from premature babies to chubby toddlers. Look for meetings of cloth diaper advocacy groups where you can discuss washable options and take a look at different types while meeting like-minded parents.

Many green families use diaper-washing services that deliver a set of freshly laundered cotton diapers to the door each week and take away the soiled ones. This type of service generally costs more than washing your own (about the same price you would spend on disposables per week). It may also use less energy than your washing machine and spares you doing the laundry.

Realistically, there may be times you find it is not practical to use a washable diaper. Completely biodegradable disposables are the latest development in green diapers. They look and work like regular disposables, but are made up of layers of unbleached cellulose filled with minimal amounts of absorbent gel and renewable absorbents, such as starch. Some biodegradable disposables are guaranteed free from harmful dioxins and chemicals such as formaldehyde, and suit babies with eczema. These diapers are highly biodegradable, but only in an earthworm composter; they don't decompose as easily if you discard them into waste that ends up in a landfill.

It takes 3.5 times
more energy
to manufacture disposable
rather than reusable diapers

CLEANSING LOTION

This all-natural baby cleansing lotion can take the place of baby wipes: spritz it onto fair-trade unbleached cotton balls or washable cloths, and use it to clean your baby's bottom at diaper changes.

1 Pour freshly boiled water into a tea-pot containing two organic chamomile tea bags—if you prefer, you can use a loose-leaf chamomile infusion instead. Leave the tea to steep (and cool) for 15 minutes.

2 Put 1 tbsp hemp oil into a measuring cup and pour in about 1 cup of the warm tea. If your baby is over one year old, add 1 tsp pasteurized clear honey and whisk well to combine the oil and honey.

3 Fill a clean, reusable glass bottle with a spray-pump almost to the top with cooled tea. Screw on the top and shake well to combine all the ingredients. Use immediately, or, once completely cool, store the bottle in the refrigerator.

4 At diaper-change time, spray a little of the lotion onto a cotton ball or a cloth wipe, then use to clean your baby's bottom. Repeat as necessary. Make up a new batch of lotion every few days and keep refrigerated.

MAKING THE CHANGE

The washable diaper system consists of three main components, which you can buy or borrow: the main diaper, the liner, and the waterproof outer wrap.

What you need

- **Main diaper**—try several shapes and sizes to see which best suits your baby (your local "real diaper" group can help; see p.186). You'll need about 24 diapers.

- **Liners**— if you are feeling conscientious, use washable liners. You may want to use a cotton or silk booster-liner for extra security, at night, or while your baby is tiny. Four to six will be plenty. Flushable, fully biodegradable paper liners are useful for disposing of solid waste.

- **Outer wrap**—this keeps everything together and protects clothing from leaks. You'll need about four.

- **Extras**—if the diapers don't have velcro or poppers, diaper fasteners are useful. You'll also need a diaper pail with a lid, and a tote bag to carry everything in.

diaper   **liner**   **outer wrap**

CHANGING A WASHABLE DIAPER

The actual method of changing a reusable diaper is
almost identical to that of a disposable, except that
there are a few more components to deal with.

1 Lay your baby on the changing mat. Remove the dirty
diaper. Put the booster liner (if using) and the diaper
into the diaper pail, and then flush the paper liner away. Put
the diaper wrap to one side. Add 2 tsp bicarbonate of soda to
the pail and fill with water, then put on the lid.

2 Lifting your baby's feet in one hand, wipe her bottom
using fair-trade unbleached organic cotton balls or
an unbleached cotton washable wipe or muslin square
dampened with water only. Discard the cotton balls or place
the dirty wipe into the diaper pail. Pat your baby's bottom
dry with a muslin square. If needed, smear on a thin layer
of an organic diaper cream to prevent diaper rash.

3 Place a clean booster liner (if using) inside a clean
diaper and fold. Lay the flushable liner on top. Slide
under your baby by lifting her feet, then secure the diaper
using the diaper fasteners.

4 Adjust the fasteners of the outer wrap to ensure a snug
fit over the diaper.

The green, clean baby: Greener diapers

Eco diaper solutions

Many parents use a mix of green diaper systems, using compostable disposables at night or when out and about, and washables at home.

The secret to keeping reusable diapers green is not to wash them at too high a temperature. Try washing mostly at 105°F (40°C), with a little eco-laundry detergent or laundry-balls. Avoid regular detergents; many contain optical brighteners, and fabric conditioner, too: both stick to fabric, making it less absorbent and more likely to cause a rash. Gentle handwashing is the best way to deal with woolen outer wraps (though felted wool can be machine-washed on a cold-water wool setting). You don't have to wash these too often, since the lanolin in wool is naturally antibacterial. Avoid putting washable diapers and their outer wraps in the dryer; it can shrink and shred the fabric, causing the waterproof wraps to disintegrate. Dry outdoors whenever possible—sunlight is a powerful bleaching agent.

The greenest "diaper" option might make you gasp: not to use diapers at all, a technique used in many parts of the world. Known as elimination communication or timing, this involves tuning in with your baby's routine, and noticing her gestures and facial and verbal expressions when she is about to go to the bathroom (so you can catch it in a potty!). Advocates value the intimacy and mutual responsiveness this method establishes.

light green Use disposables that really are disposable: compostable eco-diapers (don't forget to compost the packaging, too). Look into setting up a home composting system using earthworms (vermicomposting). Or there may be a program that picks up from your door for central earthworm composting. Avoid encasing these diapers in diaper bags (biodegradable or not).

mid green Use washable diapers and have them washed by a diaper service. Alternatively, wash them yourself with an eco-laundry detergent in the washing machine. If the diapers are secondhand, give yourself a pat on the back, and keep hanging them out to dry (rather than putting them in the dryer) so that they last long enough to pass on to another baby.

deep green Join the diaper-free movement by avoiding diapers as often as you can, and embracing elimination timing before your baby is six months old. The benefits are obvious—no diapers, no extra washing, no detergents, no diaper-rash creams, and perhaps best of all, no cost! Many one-year-olds whose parents use this method are fully potty-trained in their second year.

Green nursery: a safer space to sleep and grow

Green sleep options

Don't be disheartened if, after spending time and money decorating a baby's room the eco way, you find her sharing your room for the first few months. This can be the greenest option of all, since it uses the fewest resources.

Sound sleeping boosts immunity naturally in babies and exhausted parents

Does your baby even need a separate room? Studies suggest that babies who sleep in a crib in the same room as their parents for the first six months of life have a reduced risk of SIDS (sudden infant death syndrome). Some parents like to take this further and share their *bed* with the baby, and research finds that babies who sleep this way wake less in the night and settle back to sleep more quickly. Many breastfeeding mothers swear that this method of sleeping makes night feedings a breeze, and studies back this up—although breastfed babies who sleep with their mothers feed more often, they disturb their mothers less. However, a 2004 study found that this method of sleeping, known as co-sleeping, slightly increased the risk of SIDS.

Healthcare providers therefore insist on a few rules: no cigarettes, alcohol, or drugs that make you drowsy, and think again if you have a sleep disorder, such as sleep apnea, or if your baby was premature or small at birth. It's advised that you make a safe space for the baby at the top of the mattress, with no pillows and her own bedding; check that there are no gaps between the head of the bed and the wall or headboard. Dress your baby lightly, since beds with lots of people in them get hot (to check her temperature, touch her tummy). You might be less cramped if you invest in a crib that abuts the parental bed (see p.121), so your baby has her own safe space and bedding, and you can relax rather than trying not to move all night. This arrangement is safer if you're not around, too, as you won't always want to go to bed at the same time as your baby.

Most older babies do move into their own room, and many parents report that their baby sleeps better without the distraction of grown-ups, who may themselves welcome the freedom to read, talk, or even enjoy uninhibited sex. Don't rush out to buy a baby monitor once your baby sleeps alone (unless you live in a mansion or your baby has a chronic breathing problem). You may disturb your baby's sleep if you rush in to check on every cough.

If your baby's erratic sleep pattern is getting you down, talk to your healthcare provider. You might also like to visit a cranial osteopath or homeopath, or investigate baby sleep clinics that specialize in natural methods of sleep-training.

Green nursery: Green sleep options

NATURAL SOOTHING

Try these naturally soothing strategies instead of relying on sleep-inducing electronic gadgets, such as self-rocking cradles or teddy bears with a heartbeat.

Baby sleeping strategies

- **Darkness**—being exposed to complete darkness at night and to outdoor light in the day seems to correlate with better sleep (and growth in premature babies). Under-twos who sleep with a light on may be more likely to be nearsighted.
- **Constant noise**—many babies sleep better with regular household noise or music rather than complete silence.
- **Swaddling**—this makes tiny babies feel secure.

- **Ambient temperature**—aim for a room heated to 68°F (20°C) with bedding of one sheet and two layers of blanket.
- **Daytime naps**—babies who take routine naps during the day seem to sleep better at night than those who don't.
- **A set bedtime**—whether your baby seems sleepy or not: some infants become more lively the more tired they are.
- **Bedtime routine**—a consistent ritual (such as milk, bath, story, cuddle, singing) teaches a baby to anticipate sleep.
- **Put your baby to bed still awake**—he'll learn to drift off without you and then do so again if he wakes in the night.

To swaddle your baby, lie him on a wrap, then fold one side across his body, tucking the excess under his arm; repeat on the other side.

CRIBS AND BASKETS

During the first three years, a baby spends more time asleep than awake, so where he sleeps is an especially important consideration in your green home.

Your baby's first sleeping place might be a bassinet next to your bed rather than a full-sized crib in her own room. These baskets are made of biodegradable, renewable materials, such as palm and wicker. If a basket your baby will grow out of within weeks seems like an unnecessary expense (and a waste of resources), borrow one, or choose a sturdy wicker version to use later as a toy basket or doll's bed. Look for baskets made from renewable local materials, with handles for carrying. Although regular infant carriers are another cozy option, they tend to be made of plastic, especially if part of a stroller or playpen, and may require a separate mattress for nighttime. Wooden cribs tend to last longer than bassinets, but they aren't as readily portable. You might like to try a cheap, fully recyclable eco-crib made of cardboard, which is easy to assemble and reassemble for nights away from home, but do ask how it achieves its fire retardance and consider its durability.

Hammocks have been an infant's ideal first bed for centuries in many cultures. As the baby moves, he gently rocks himself, and the fabric cocoons him in womblike security, while supporting his head in a position that may help to prevent reflux.

Green nursery: Green sleep options

Hammocks can be soothing for colicky babies and also prevent infants from rolling onto their fronts (supine is the recommended sleeping position to reduce the risk of SIDS). Specially designed baby hammocks are used in neonatal intensive care units in hospitals around the world because of these unique features.

When choosing a crib, look for features that extend its life span, such as a removable side that allows the crib to abut the parental bed or a design that turns into a toddler bed or sofa. Solid wood from managed, renewable sources is best. Ask suppliers about nontoxic varnishes and finishes rather than synthetic sealants: your baby will soon start chewing the bars.

In two US studies, only organic cotton crib mattresses had no toxic emissions

Mattresses are an especially important eco consideration, whether for a bassinet or a crib, since most readily available mattresses are made from polyurethane foam and PVC. Both harm the environment in their manufacture and disposal, and may emit noxious gases such as toluene or styrene, or fire retardants shown to interfere with infant brain development. Natural mattresses are harder to source and more expensive, but much longer-lasting and better for the environment. Look for those made from natural latex, coir (from coconut shells), and pure new wool, with an organic cotton cover. Natural fibers wick away moisture from the body, helping to maintain a more even temperature all night long. Natural and organic mattresses are also made from materials that meet fire-safety compliance standards without being treated with fire-retardant chemicals; these build up in the body and have been linked with childhood learning and behavioral problems.

Cribs and mattresses are costly to purse and planet, so conserve both by sourcing them secondhand. Although studies have linked toxic bacteria in used mattresses with SIDS, the UK-based Foundation for the Study of Infant Deaths states that any mattress is OK as long as it's firm, not sagging, and doesn't show wear and tear. First, consider these factors:

Secondhand crib safety checklist

- Reject cribs with cracks, broken slats, cut-out decorations, or protruding bolts or posts. Look for a JPMA certification.
- Space between bars must be less than 2⅜ in (60 mm).
- Avoid if the base isn't firm or the sides don't lock upright.
- Check for peeling paint and avoid pre-1980s painted cribs.
- Make sure the mattress fits snugly on all four sides.
- Does the mattress have a top layer you can detach to wash at 140°F (60°C)? If not, vacuum well to kill dust mites.

Bassinets are ideal for very young babies because they are highly portable and make your baby feel snug and secure.

Green nursery: Green sleep options

Asthma and allergic conditions
are associated primarily

with exposure to

indoor contaminants

Regular mattresses may be treated with **fire retardants**

that can affect brain function

GREEN BEDDING

Buying baby bedding is an eco-shopper's paradise; there's a virtual superstore of green options, from super-soft organic cotton to silk.

Organic cotton sheets and cellular blankets are recommended for babies under one year. Look for fair trade options, extra-soft Pima cotton, or Demeter-certified organic wool blankets. Don't be put off by the ivory color; it shows that the fabric hasn't been treated with harsh chlorine bleach. You might like an organic cotton mattress pad if using a secondhand or conventional mattress. Bamboo is an even more eco-friendly option for sheets, since it is softer, more hypoallergenic, and stays drier than cotton.

Many parents prefer baby sleeping bags to sheets and blankets. Put your baby to bed in his sleeper and a bag suitable for the season (they vary in thickness). Bags are great for wriggly babies—they can enjoy having a good kick, but can't kick off the covers, so they stay snug all night (which means less night waking for all of you). Look for bags made from organic cotton or soft merino wool, which adjusts naturally to the temperature of the baby and the room.

In your baby's second year (but not before), he might like to have an organic cotton pillow and a comforter or duvet. Organic wool and silk are the best comforter options for temperature control, and are naturally hypoallergenic.

Green nursery: Green sleep options

Eco bedding solutions

Baby sleeping bags, blankets, swaddling robes—
with so many bedding options to choose from,
how do you select the greenest choice?

The push to produce cheap textiles in the last decade has led to
some unethical trade practices, including sweatshop conditions
and child labor. How can you avoid supporting this? Choosing
certified organic goods is a good start, but not the whole story,
since this only guarantees the raw ingredients. To be sure that
the weaving and manufacturing of fabric is as ethical as its
growing, look for the SKAL logo, a sign of ethical textile
processing, or the Oeko-Tex mark, which indicates that processing
practices have minimal environmental impact and that products
are of high quality (its standards for baby clothes are more
stringent than for other textiles). You might also look for the FWF
(Fair Wear Foundation) logo, which shows that textiles have
been produced in fair-labor conditions; those marked "fair trade"
only certify that producers were given a fair wage for the raw
material, and don't cover processing and manufacturing stages.

At home, try to buy from small local producers. The best
might buy wool from farmers who struggle to make a profit from
traditional farming, then employ women with skills that are fast
being lost to knit clothes and blankets using traditional patterns
and techniques, preserving our heritage for future generations.

light green Buy brand-new, unbleached, certified organic cotton sheets and you can reassure yourself that few artificial fertilizers and pesticides were used by those who farm the crops. This protects the soil and water sources, as well as the health of the farmer and his family. And you can guarantee that your baby won't spend hours lying on fabric that contains pesticide residues.

mid green Borrow, or buy secondhand if you can't borrow, an organic cotton baby sleeping bag or two (a lightweight version for summer and a warmer one for winter), then forget about top sheets or blankets. Merino wool bags require less washing (simply air them outdoors), but if your baby is allergy-prone, choose one that can be washed at 140°F (60°C) to kill dust mites.

deep green Get Grandma to knit a baby blanket from wool from local sheep farmers, or ask friends to meet up for a knitting evening to knit a square each to sew into a baby blanket, or to patchwork cotton fabric remnants into a quilt (not suitable for young babies). Look for vintage linen sheets at antique textile fairs woven from plants raised before the days of pesticides; they're likely to be of good quality.

Decorating baby's room

The urge to nest has many of us stripping walls, sanding floors, and redecorating before a baby arrives. But you need to protect your baby's health and the environment.

When you're pregnant or have a small baby, don't stay at home while rooms are being sanded or stripped of old paint; the dust may contain hazardous toxins, such as lead, which was added to paint until the 1970s. It's best to have someone else do the dirty work and clean up afterward, and to get major work done well in advance of the baby's arrival. Wait for a few weeks and air a newly decorated room very well before allowing a baby to sleep in it. A new paint smell indicates the presence of the climate-changing chemicals known as VOCs (volatile organic compounds). These chemical solvents include toluene, exposure to which increases the risk of neurological and developmental problems. VOCs also trigger headaches and have been associated with postpartum depression. They are off-gassed by paint for years. Recent EU regulations have resulted in fewer VOCs in paint, but also in the addition of dangerous replacement chemicals, such as ammonia, acetone, and biocides, and more energy-intensive production processes. How do you choose a better paint? Avoid those made by multinational chemical companies (i.e., most paints in home improvement stores). Buy instead from small manufacturers that specialize in natural paint, declare their environmental standards, and list the ingredients on the can. Most eco-paints are low in VOCs or have none at all, and have fewer synthetic chemicals than regular paints.

Carpets and PVC-backed flooring are the second-most-potent source of toxins at home after paint. If you can, remove them completely from a baby's room. If you don't like bare boards, lay linoleum (which is made from linseed oil and is

PVC flooring in a child's room is the strongest single cause of respiratory ailments

completely biodegradable), or flooring woven from bamboo or grasses (choose natural backing and have it installed the old-fashioned way—with nails, not glue). If you can't do without carpet, choose 100 percent untreated wool. It's biodegradable, naturally fire-resistant, remains soft for years, and even purifies the room (wool absorbs airborne contaminants such as formaldehyde, and binds them in for up to 30 years). Wool is hypoallergenic; research suggests it resists dust mites more effectively than nylon carpet.

FURNISHING YOUR BABY'S ROOM

Once you've redecorated your baby's room, you'll want to add nontoxic, environmentally-friendly furnishings that will last.

Think about the big furniture first—an armoire or chest for storing baby clothing and toys, diapers, and changing materials; perhaps a toddler-sized table and chairs; a rocking chair for feeding; and a bookshelf. Question whether you need a changing table; you're unlikely to use it after the first year, and it's safer to change your child on the floor on a plastic-free changing mat. Green shoppers opt for solid wood furniture from forests managed sustainably. The FSC certification stamp guarantees that the wood in your furniture can be traced back to a forest managed in an environmentally responsible and socially beneficial way. Also consider wooden items made from newer green materials, such as bamboo or coconut. It's greener still to buy furniture made from reclaimed lumber, and greenest of all to fill your home with "pre-loved" furniture—buying secondhand

Green nursery: Decorating your baby's room

Every day in the US, about
15,000 tons
of discarded wood are
chipped or sent to landfill

saves trees and energy, and makes your home look unique in an era of cheap, fashion-led furnishing. Buying locally sourced and made pieces saves wood miles, too. Most furniture has a high carbon footprint because it's so bulky to transport.

Chemical-free is the only way to go with babies, so avoid composite-wood furniture, which is manufactured by gluing together thin slices of wood with adhesives that may contain (and off-gas) formaldehyde and other chemical nasties. Avoid also anything that might have been varnished with synthetic chemicals. To be extra-sure furniture won't off-gas VOCs, look for items made the old-fashioned way, using mortise-and-tenon joints—no glues or even screws or nails. Custom eco-furniture designed and made locally may be high in price, but if you buy just one piece you adore, you're more likely to cherish and preserve it for many years, which you might not do with a flimsy self-assembled item—and this saves money (in the long-term) as well as the planet. If you're ditching old furniture, look for an organization that will repair and redistribute it, rather than taking it to the dump.

Instead of rushing out to buy all-new eco curtains, pillows, and rugs, see what you can revamp and customize from elsewhere. Then search out furnishing fabrics in organic cotton, robust hemp, or jute. Reserve a good part of your budget for thick-lined curtains that keep out the light and keep in warmth. Draw them at dusk to save money on heating bills.

Hemp is a particularly effective insulating material, said to have the best heat-ratio capacity of any natural fiber. It also resists fading from light. When buying fabric to make your own curtains, ask about the chemicals used to print and dye it, and decline finishes such as permanent pressing and stain-guards, which may coat the fabric in chemicals thought to damage immunity and reproductive hormones. PVC blackout backing is another no-no. As well as damaging the environment with chlorine and dioxins, studies link PVC and its plasticizing chemicals with childhood respiratory problems and asthma.

The all-natural soft furnishing your baby will love most is a lambskin for luxurious lounging. As ever, choose local and unbleached if you can; some skins are tanned with mimosa rather than harsh chemicals, others might be guaranteed free from organophosphates (nerve agents used in sheep-dip) or heavy metals used in conventional tanning. Buying direct from a farm guarantees income for sheep farmers, and you might pick up an interesting skin from a heritage breed. They resist stains and are self-cleansing, but can be machine-washed in cool water. Lying on a lambskin (which is naturally warm in winter and cool in summer) seems to soothe babies and to encourage better sleep, greater contentment, and weight gain.

Use wooden furniture from sustainable sources and fabrics made from natural materials for your child's nursery.

Green nursery: Decorating your baby's room

Play green: natural ways to learn and have fun

The mini-consumer

It's easy to get sucked into a world of primary-colored plastic and "baby genius" toys after giving birth. Here's how and why to resist the pressure.

Even before a baby is born, the pressure's on for us to brand her room, wardrobe, and toy box with the licensed characters of movies and TV. This helps to create a throwaway mentality and acquisitive brand awareness from birth, since each new set of merchandise makes the last one obsolete. Aggressive marketing targets parents and children, driving the consumer mill. Why is this bad for the planet as well as our children's health? Manufacturing, transportation, and disposal (most toys are made from petrochemicals in China and can't be recycled) all eat up ancient forest and fossil fuels and emit climate-change gases. Worries center around PVC, one of the forms of plastic most often used in toy-making; when made or incinerated, PVC emits dioxins—carcinogens that build up in soil, water, food, and our bodies. Health concerns also surround the plasticizing chemicals that make PVC soft, especially phthalates, which may easily leach out—Danish studies on teething rings found "significant migration" of phthalates. Initial studies link them with damage to the reproductive system, kidneys, and liver, and also to asthma. The US Environment Protection Agency regards one phthalate, called DEHP, as a "probable human carcinogen."

So concerned is the European Union that in January 2007 it banned three phthalates (DEHP, DBP, BBP) from toys and childcare products in concentrations of more than 0.1 percent. Three more (DINP, DIDP, DNOP) were banned from any toys that under-threes put in their mouths. Other potentially dangerous additives in plastic toys include organotins (which can disrupt testosterone), nonylphenol (can damage immunity), and the toxic heavy metals cadmium and lead. Some toys for the very young have tested positive for harmful fire retardants. But don't dump Barbie; she might leach toxins into landfills or into the air if incinerated. Don't recycle her either. Not all toys are marked with a plastic number (only those numbered "2", "4", or "5" can be recycled) and those without spoil all the plastic in a batch.

Research shows that children as young as 18 months old can recognize brands

You are probably not responsible for the pile of plastic toys suffocating your mini-consumer. Most likely, they rain in from adoring friends and family. Why not suggest that the best gift of all is for these people to spend time with your child—to take her to the park, a toddler swim session, or a puppet show. When stuff is so omnipresent, giving time is a thoughtful way to show love.

Play green: The mini-consumer

By one estimate, in 2007 some **17 million** imported **toys** from China were **recalled** because of **lead contamination**— and most will end up in **landfills**

Manufacture of toys

Many green parents like to consider how and where a toy was made as well as what materials it's made from.

Many toys on the market in North America are produced in China (which manufactures some 80 percent of the world's toys) on behalf of multinational companies. Though working conditions are improving, they are not ideal at many sites where working time and pay-regulation directives may not be enforced. The seasonal nature of our buying habits also has an impact, leading to periods of excessive working hours followed by unemployment. There is concern that a drop in toy prices in the past ten years (by 33 percent in the US), despite the rising prices of raw materials, is made possible by cheap labor. The trend toward cost-cutting has also been linked to the safety recall in 2007 of millions of toys made in China that had powerful detachable magnets and were contaminated with lead paint.

What can you do? Write to your favorite toy manufacturer, telling them you care about the workers who make your child's toys, and asking about measures they are taking to ameliorate conditions. If you don't get a satisfactory answer, stop buying their toys, and talk to your friends about your decision. Why not begin a blog? People underestimate consumer power, but if you let your views be known, you may be surprised at the results.

Greener toys

The good news is that toys don't have to be made of plastic, and there is a wide selection of green options available.

Naturally germ-resistant, durable, and fully degradable, wooden toys are the most obvious choice for an ethical consumer. Choose solid (not particle) wood from sustainable sources (look for the FSC logo) and check that varnishes and paints are nontoxic, water-based, and free of VOCs (volatile organic compounds). Linseed, walnut oil, and beeswax are nontoxic alternative

Natural materials make toys appealing and sustainable.

Handmade gifts have a prized place among your baby's toys.

coatings. Be vigilant about teethers and rattles: untreated natural wood may be best. Sustainable rubberwood is a good choice; it comes from trees felled at the end of their latex production life. If the wood is indigenous and the toy locally made, perhaps by people without much paid work, give yourself a big green check mark. Recycled, biodegradable cardboard toys are fun, too, even though they are designed to be thrown away.

Hemp or organic cotton cuddly toys are popular with babies. Since they get sucked and hugged to sweaty bodies, be sure the dyes are environment- and baby-friendly. Teddy bears stuffed and finished with organic wool are good for children prone to allergies, as wool deters dust mites.

Nontoxic paints are vital for toys that may be chewed.

Long-lasting toys can be passed on as family heirlooms.

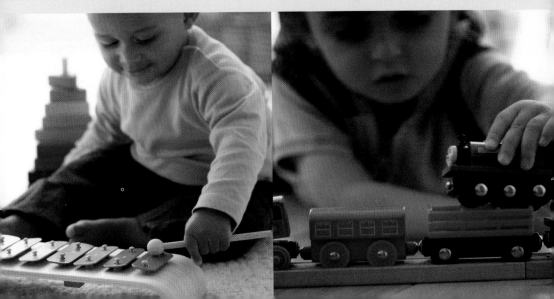

MAKING YOUR OWN TOYS

It may be hard to resist pressure to buy toys, but with a little effort you can show your child what fun it can be to improvise toys from household items.

Homemade toys tend to foster open-ended creative play—the unstructured play crucial to infant learning. Researchers find that toys that direct play, such as electronic gadgets that require children to press buttons or give right and wrong answers, may discourage creativity, undermine basic motor skills, and shorten attention span. They also set up a barrier to social interaction. To stimulate these childhood essentials, spend time together improvising toys from household objects. Make a doll from a wooden spoon by drawing on a face with nontoxic pens and tying a fabric dress around its "neck." As your baby grows, graduate to homemade clothespin dolls and rag dolls. Throw together a dress-up box of cast-offs and cut-downs. Make your own play dough (search online for a recipe for an edible version): polymer clays contain PVC, and phthalates have been found on children's hands even after washing. The most ethical toys are your child's own fingers and toes: explore them with songs or a book of counting rhymes.

Homemade toys are fun to make, and foster your child's resourcefulness and creativity, without costing much.

MAKING A TREASURE BASKET

Natural and household objects are an easy way to encourage your baby's sensory exploration when she can sit steadily. Fill a basket with objects of varying texture, color, size, and shape.

1 First, look for hard objects. They must be large enough to handle and suck without risk of swallowing. Try smooth pebbles, shells, and twigs; shiny surfaces, such as metal cups; objects for threading (like wooden curtain rings), or that stack inside each other (like Russian dolls).

2 Now find soft objects: long, clean feathers, a leather key fob, sheep's wool, leaves; fabrics such as velvet, silk, linen, and felt (make them into bags to put objects into and take out); small wicker baskets for sorting like with like.

3 Add some natural scents: a lavender bag or pine cones; or put cinnamon sticks or vanilla pods in a spice-shaker. Create noise with coconut shells, jingling metal bangles, a bunch of keys, or hand bells.

4 Stay with your baby while she explores her treasures, ask what happens if she shakes or smells them, and add new items regularly to keep her interest alive.

Play green: Greener toys

SECONDHAND TOYS

"Share and repair" is the mantra for green parents—and one worth passing on to your children. When you want a new toy for your child, just think secondhand.

Because we buy so many toys, there is a huge number of unwanted quality toys in circulation. Instead of buying brand new, start your search at garage sales and charity shops, and browse newspaper classifieds and Freecycle postings. Try secondhand baby shops, which vet toys for safety. If you don't find what you want, go global with online auction sites.

Supporting secondhand exchange is a two-way transaction. Rather than discarding toys your child has grown out of, find them a new home. Sort through the toy box before birthdays or Christmas, and bag up items your child has outgrown before the next deluge arrives. Sort them into three piles: one to put away as heirlooms or keepsakes, or pass on to siblings and cousins; one to sell online or at a yard sale; and one to donate to a charity shop, hospital, doctor's office, or daycare. Encourage toddlers to help; it makes the task longer and potentially tearful, but it starts them thinking about the worth of objects and what happens to stuff they no longer need. Some manufacturers of large toys, such as plastic kitchens or garden equipment, take back items for recycling. Try out a toy library, if there's one in your area, where you can borrow new toys every week for free and socialize with other parents.

Long-lasting secondhand buys include collections that can be added to, for constant rekindling of the urge to play, and durable solid wood and metal objects. What's best avoided? Take the sniff test; if a toy smells like new plastic, it's full of phthalates. Don't buy pre-1980s painted items (may contain lead), toys with fluid or electronic components, and damaged goods.

Even ethical toys stop being ethical if they end up discarded in a landfill site

Covetable secondhand toys

- **Lego**—indestructible and free of phthalates; no-PVC policy.
- **Playmobil**—for older toddlers; no-PVC policy.
- **Käthe Kruse dolls**—handcrafted dolls made of wood and cloth that can be repaired in the German factory.
- **Brio train set**—choose wood, though all Brio is PVC-free.
- **IKEA toys**—all are free of PVC and iffy woods and dyes.
- **Wooden dollhouse, fort, or puppet theater**—collecting the accessories and dolls separately adds to the adventure.
- **Metal construction toys**—durable and can be added to.

CLEANING TOYS

Involve your toddler in cleaning and repairing her own toys and she will learn very early that good care and mending lengthen the life span of her favorite things.

Cleaning toys can be a fun activity to do together. Lay newspaper on the floor or work outdoors, then fill one bowl with warm soapy water (use an eco dishwashing liquid) and another with plain warm water. You'll also need two wooden scrub brushes, dishcloths, and dry towels. Dump the toys in the soapy water and scrub well, then rinse in the clean water, and dry with a towel. Hang up doll clothes or soft toys to dry outdoors. It's best to avoid bleach or antibacterial soap, wipes, and sprays. Antibacterial cleaners are no more effective than soap and water, and may contain the antimicrobial pesticide triclosan (highly toxic if it enters the marine environment). They may also contain denatured ethanol, an irritant to eyes and mucous membranes. The residue from sprays lingers on surfaces and toys, ready to transfer to tiny fingers and mouths.

   To rid soft toys and woolen items of dust mites and wool moths, place them in a plastic bag and freeze for a few days, then machine-wash with eco washing powder at 140°F (60°C), or 85°F (30°C) for wool, and hang up to dry outside.

Getting wet is all part of the fun when your toddler helps to keep his toys clean.

Play green: Greener toys

Eco toy solutions

There are so many environment-friendly toys available that it's easy to slip into an unethical shopping fest and buy too much. The greenest rule of toy-buying might be to buy nothing at all!

To be sure that the toy manufacturers you buy from have ethical practices, only buy toys made in the US or Canada, or from fair trade projects. Plastic toys from outside North America may contain banned or restricted phthalates, and it's tricky to tell if they do because so many aren't marked with a plastic number. The most ethical way to buy new toys is to choose soft toys and solid wooden toys handcrafted locally. They might not be organic or use recycled materials, but they cut down on toy miles, allow you to opt out of multinational trading if you find it distasteful, and, importantly, present your child with something original. Offering an alternative to mass-market products may help offset the anxiety children can suffer when involved in consumer culture.

In the end, if every moment becomes a green shopping or learning opportunity, even ethical toys become just another part of the same consumer pressure. The greenest act of all is not to buy or acquire anything for a while and instead to spend time with your baby with no objects at all. Rather than guiding this free-play session, simply look at your baby and react to her prompts as she sets the agenda for what you do.

light green Buy a fair-trade toy, such as the educational toys produced by families in Sri Lanka for Lanka Kada: this project supplies year-round employment and cuts out middlemen. Such producers tend to avoid PVC and excess packaging, as they do not want to waste resources. Buying a fair-trade toy for your baby means that it was not been made in a sweatshop by another child.

mid green Play with Lego. As it's made of plastic, it might seem a curious eco-choice, but children play with it for around ten years and it's durable enough to pass down the generations. Second-hand Lego is rare, proof of how highly parents and kids rate it. Unlike most plastic toys, it doesn't emit noxious fumes and the manufacturer has impressive waste- and energy-minimizing policies.

deep green Make a playhouse from a cardboard box. Cut holes for windows and doors, then play peekaboo, a toxin-free, eco-friendly way to entertain infants. When your baby gets bored, tear it up and compost or send it off in your curbside collection. Make another a month or two later. Or sew your own soft toy from cast-offs, stuffing it with scraps of fabric. There are no rules; let your imagination take flight.

Introducing books

Babies who "read" books with their parents tend to demonstrate enhanced language skills, focus, motivation, and concentration, and have a head-start in reading when they go to school.

However, a 2007 study found that primary-school children spend twice as long watching TV as reading with an adult. To cut your family's future carbon footprint, start the reading habit young and thus reduce TV use—you can introduce your baby to colorful picture books from birth. She may become so excited by the activity that within a few months she'll be batting the pages of favorite board books in her eagerness to get to the next picture. Read books of rhymes and lullabies with your baby, too. Nursery rhymes are especially good because they imprint rhythms and sound patterns in your baby's brain that mirror those of speech. Books also help your baby to learn how to listen. Reading may be as valuable for bonding as for brain development because it's something you do together; sharing a book is a special time of cosy one-to-one interaction.

Join your local **library,** one of the most enjoyable ways to reuse and **recycle**

Unlike other forms of entertainment, like watching TV or listening to music, you can't read and do anything else at the same time. Intensify the bonding process by setting aside a few minutes for reading at the same time every day, and by making the space really cozy. Sit in a comfortable chair and snuggle your baby into your lap. She'll soon begin to associate books with relaxation, which may be why reading makes such a calming addition to a bedtime routine. When reading to a baby, put on a sing-song voice, adopt funny voices for different characters, and improvise your own details (you don't have to stick to the printed text). Point out pictures with your finger. If you find any of this difficult or embarrassing, see if there's a baby book group at your local library. The children's librarian can help to build your confidence. Join the library while you're there for an endless, inherently green supply of new books.

What about educational DVDs specially engineered to boost your baby's intelligence? The hard sell might make you feel guilty if you don't use them. If you prefer to cut your carbon footprint and keep the TV off, you'll be reassured by a University of Washington study that found a large and statistically significant reduction in vocabulary among infants aged 8–16 months who watched baby DVDs or videos. Other research into babies and language development found that electronic tools weren't as effective in promoting early literacy as sharing a book, and led to a "severely truncated" reading experience.

Play green: Introducing books

CHOOSING GREENER BOOKS

Your baby will suck any book she can grasp, so if you can, choose those that are less toxic. The publishing industry is beginning to tackle environmental concerns and bring us greener books.

The greenest books are "eco-printed" using nonmetal inks on 100 percent post-consumer recycled chlorine-free paper, with presses that minimize solvent use or don't require copper plates. Green printers may also use renewable energy in printing and shipping. But these kinds of books can be hard to find.

Key features of green books

- **FSC certification**—this shows that the paper has been sourced from responsibly managed forests. Choose paper with at least 50 percent post-consumer recycled content.
- **Greener inks**—look for soy- and vegetable-based inks.
- **Water-based glues**—books with less adhesive are safer.
- **Less bleaching**—choose books that are processed chlorine-free (PCF), which substitute oxygen-based compounds instead.
- **Avoid plastic**—it might be wise to avoid bath books altogether. They tend to be made from nonrenewable petrochemicals made flexible with phthalates.

Read about the environment with your baby from the start, and he'll grow up eager to preserve it.

Play green: Introducing books

We **waste** an estimated one billion dollars' worth of **electricity** each year by leaving the TV and electronic gadgets on **standby**

Minimizing energy use

To cut your baby's carbon emissions and
production of toxic waste, say "no" to toys
with batteries or transformers.

Batteries are an all-around hassle, whether you hate the
noise of battery-operated toys, find buying new ones a constant
nuisance, worry about old batteries corroding, or just don't know
how to dispose of them. If we can't replace batteries (say, because
they're encased within fluffy creatures), or get tired of the expense
of doing so, toys lose their appeal, which brings even more hassle
for the green parent—it's almost impossible to recycle battery-
operated toys, since they're made from mixed materials. Call
your local department of sanitation or municipal recycling center
to determine what recycling options are available for batteries in
your area. If you're given battery-powered toys, take them back
and exchange them for something more durable, or ask for green
alternatives, like wind-up or solar-powered toys.

Save energy by always unplugging electrical items (such as
the TV or stereo) when not in use. You can buy a power strip that
turns off the power to a number of items at the touch of one
switch, or a motivating monitor that shows how much electricity
you're using. You could also call your electric company and ask to
purchase as much of your electricity as possible from renewable
sources such as wind power and solar installations.

Out and about: introducing your baby to a greener world

Motor vehicles form the largest source of global atmospheric **pollution**

Transportation accounts for over a quarter of US CO_2 emissions

Transporting your baby

Motor vehicles use a third of the world's oil, so how you travel makes a difference to your carbon footprint; choosing greener ways to get around can enhance your community and your baby's health.

Car use by parents is increasing more rapidly than for the rest of the population. Research suggests that this is not only because mothers' lives are increasingly complex and time-squeezed now that more of us work (and fear for our children's safety), but also because urban sprawl is increasing the distance to stores, schools, and hospitals. And taking mass transit with babies and children can be difficult and expensive. But your travel choices affect your baby's future: it seems that children who travel by car are less likely to walk to school and more likely to develop into car-dependent adults. This lack of physical activity increases the risk of heart disease, stroke, obesity, and osteoporosis.

Think about why you travel outside your neighborhood. Can you socialize, shop, and take baby classes closer to home to cut pollution and get to know your local community? When venturing afield on public transportation, travel outside of rush hours, and take a friend to handle stroller and bags or help entertain a wriggly baby. Email your bus company about making travel with a baby easier and using hybrid/biodiesel buses to make cities cleaner.

Out and about: Transporting your baby

BABY CARRIERS

Carrying infants in a sling is the ultimate in green transportation, whether they snuggle in close as tiny babies or ride high on your back as toddlers.

Slings have far less impact on the environment than any stroller or car seat, since they tend to be made of small amounts of cloth and few plastics or metals. They are not bulky to transport and are often made locally rather than being shipped around the globe. Baby carriers pass on easily from baby to baby without having to be safety-checked. Even better, slings seem to boost bonding and well-being. A study of babies carried for about three hours a day showed that they cried less, spent more time quiet and alert, and fed more often than non-carried babies. The physical stimulation and increased interaction that come with sling use may also boost growth and development, counter baby blues, and make you feel more confident as a parent. And they're certainly easier to take on a bus or train than strollers.

The greenest sling is one you make yourself (find a pattern online), but if you plan to borrow or buy one, try out a few (they all feel very different) at a secondhand baby store or organic baby shop. Look for a design that spreads weight evenly across

A versatile sling that can be used to carry a baby or toddler in a range of positions will give you the longest usage. Make sure the straps are wide enough to spread weight evenly.

your back and shoulders. The types that get used longest allow you to carry a sleeping baby lying sideways and to breastfeed discreetly, and they accommodate infants facing either inward or out, as well as toddlers on the hip and back. Organic, washable fabric is best. If possible, find out whether the sling you like has been made according to ethical working practices.

Which way should your baby face? It may be best to carry young babies facing inward, snuggled into your chest. The splayed-hip position of many slings may help strengthen the hip joints. Facing inward boosts interaction, too, helping your baby learn communication and language skills. Fussing babies, however, may like the distraction of facing outward, though the rush of stimuli can be overwhelming. Older babies often enjoy a more structured frame backpack, which suits leisure walking thanks to its extra support. The longer you carry your child, the more he gets used to pedestrian transportation, and the less likely to become a car-dependent adult. And you'll be a great role model for the benefits of exercise.

Babies who are carried seem to cry and fuss less in the first 3 months of life

CARRIAGES & STROLLERS

Trips of less than two miles (about three kilometers) are perfect for going for a spin with a stroller or baby carriage.

However, choosing a carriage can be stressful given the many options. Standard or all-terrain stroller? Travel system that morphs from car seat to stroller? Forward- or backward-facing seat? Consumer studies find that most parents prefer something that's lightweight to carry and fold (especially if you often use mass transit) and fits easily in the trunk of the car. Longevity is a good green measure—the best choice being one item that can take you from newborn to age four. Resource-intensive overengineering is to be avoided: do you really need a cup-holder or all-terrain rubber tires if you only push to the local park?

Carriages can seem bulky and old-school, but have advantages. They force you to walk, since they don't pack into a car or travel well on buses, and have space for shopping bags. Your baby can stretch out flat (essential for newborns), nap comfortably, and, perhaps most importantly, face you. Some organizations claim that forward-facing buggies hamper a baby's developing communication skills, since he can't read your face and sounds. They also place your baby at the level of car exhausts. A carriage that elevates your baby to waist height or above is healthier for your baby. The first generation of eco-buggies are lined with wool and organic cotton and free from

Out and about: Transporting your baby

PVC and chemical treatments. A vintage carriage might be even greener: built to last, they often pass down the generations. Borrow one, then buy your own at six months, once you know what suits you. Some options allow a baby to face you, then swivel to face forward as he grows. Travel systems that morph from car seat to stroller to carrier tend to be so unwieldy that parents ditch them for a lightweight stroller and a car seat that fits a growing baby. Another problem with travel systems is that babies are so portable that it's all too easy to leave them clipped in for hours as you move from car to stroller to grocery cart. Free your baby well before two hours have elapsed and don't let him sleep in a car seat for long periods: it's not great for developing bodies to be upright (encased in plastic) for hours. Flat-head syndrome, a distortion of the cranium, is becoming more common and may result from strapping babies upright for long periods. This position may also harm the spine and can lead to vomiting, low levels of blood oxygen, and breathing difficulties. The American Academy of Pediatrics advises that young babies spend minimal time in car seats (and strollers, swings, or bouncy seats). Release your baby, cuddle him, gently stretch his limbs, put him on his front or your lap, and talk face to face—or use a sling.

A stroller that converts from single to double by adding a seat attachment is ideal for the growing green family.

BUYING SECONDHAND

Sales of brand-new baby goods, from slings and other carriers to strollers and car seats, are at an all-time high. It seems we have gotten out of the habit of passing on and buying secondhand. But it really is a much greener option.

Studies attribute the trend for buying new, in part, to the pressure from trade associations, an argument that is often presented as a matter of safety. However, it's quite safe to purchase and borrow sturdy used carriages and strollers if you follow a few rules:

Secondhand safety points

- Check that the brakes hold the carriage or stroller securely on a slope.
- Check that the wheels seem securely fixed and undamaged.
- The folding action should be smooth and controlled by two separate locks, with no parts or sharp edges to trap fingers.
- Look at the harness; it should have a five-point action (fitting over the shoulders, around the waist, and through the legs). Check that you can adjust the fit of the straps.
- Can you remove fabric to wash it, or replace accessories to extend the life of the carriage or stroller?

Out and about: Transporting your baby

For car seats, the standard advice is always to buy new and make sure your chosen model meets current federal safety standards. However, many green parents feel happy inheriting used seats if they are fairly new (and so likely to meet current safety standards) and come from a trusted source, who can guarantee that the car seat has not been involved in an accident. Even if you can guarantee the provenance of a used seat, it's vital to examine it for damage (although you won't be able to see interior damage). It's also important to have the original instructions to be able to install the seat correctly. Consider having the installed seat checked by a certified child passenger safety technician, to be sure it fits both car and child correctly. Decline any seat if it won't fit your car snugly or is not appropriate for your child's age and weight. When buying a new car seat, check the manufacturer's website for their policy on using cadmium or lead, bromine or chlorine, phthalates, or PVC—if they don't have a policy, it might be sensible to avoid their products. You might like to make a cover in organic cotton to fit over nonorganic car seats.

NHTSA studies suggest that **82% of car seats** are installed and used **incorrectly**

Out and about: Transporting your baby

TRAVELING BY BICYCLE

Cycling, the second most green mode of transportation after walking, is enjoying a renaissance worldwide; so don't feel you have to give up now you have a baby.

Children are essential to the future of this cycling renaissance, and may be more likely to see cycling as an alternative to car travel if they gain confidence by starting the habit young.

Babies are usually ready to start traveling on your bike once they can sit up confidently (with their head unsupported) and tolerate the weight of a helmet. For most babies this happens after their first birthday and once they reach about 20 lb (9 kg). You'll be able to keep your baby in a seat until he outgrows its weight limit (around 33 lb/15 kg or 49 lb/22 kg, depending on the seat), which may be well after his fourth birthday. There are seat options for the front, middle, and rear of an adult bike, as well as trailers that usually attach to the back. Many parents favor the rear-mounted seat, since piling weight onto the front of a bike affects the steering and balance (and a child on a bike makes the

The number of
cycle journeys
made in London has risen by
100% in 5 years

ride more unstable anyway), even if enclosing your child between your arms on a cross-bar seat feels safer. Trailers that carry one or two children are another option (some can even be converted into a stroller), but, again, babies must be able to sit upright and maintain the weight of a helmet. This option may be best on quiet streets, cycle paths, and country roads.

The most suitable bicycle for carrying or towing a child is a solid, reliable hybrid (a cross between a mountain bike and a road bike) with a good range of gears. Go for one that suits the climate and geography of your region: hilly or flat, dry or wet, salty or urban grimy. For advice, consult your bike shop, other parent cyclists, and Internet forums; they'll also have tips on regaining confidence if you haven't ridden for a while. If you plan to buy secondhand bike, take a specialist along with you to vet it.

Bike manufacturing isn't as green as in the past, when components and bikes may have been manufactured in the US and were repairable. Most bikes and components are now made and assembled in Asia, and it can be difficult (and often more than the bike is worth) to bring them up to current safety standards. Because of yearly technological advances, parts may not be compatible between models. For safety reasons, have your bike serviced every year by a reputable bike shop; if possible, choose one that recycles tires, metal, and packaging.

Out and about: Transporting your baby

BABY CYCLING EQUIPMENT

When buying new cycling gear, make an independent bike shop your first port of call, and inquire about the company's ethos and the materials used.

Make sure the staff of your chosen bike shop includes experienced cyclists and knowledgeable bike mechanics, and that current customers are happy to recommend them. To put different bikes to the test, rent them first from a bike rental shop and have a green family outing. Ask for advice on which type of seat is most appropriate for your child's age and size, the kind of bike you ride, and your region's climate and geography.

Cycle dealers say there is no sure way of finding a safe and reliable secondhand child bicycle seat. Whether you decide to buy new or secondhand, look for the ASTM 1625-00 safety standard, a five-point harness, and a footguard, and if you have doubts, ask your bike shop to check it over and advise you on installing it safely.

A helmet is something you must buy new, unless you know its history inside out. (If you have an accident, you *must* buy a new helmet.) There is a variety of sizes, pads, and adjustments, so have your baby's helmet fitted by an expert. And you might want an antipollution mask for yourself if you live in the city.

Start cycling on bike paths to brush up your cycling skills and give toddlers an exciting journey they'll love.

Out and about: Transporting your baby

Green places to go

Staying close to home has many merits when you have a baby, not least that it's greenest to travel only as far as you can walk or push.

You don't have to drive to a nature reserve to have fun introducing your baby to the natural world; it's all around you. Stroll to your local park, showing your baby the sky, birds, and insects; allow him to touch bark, soil, and crunchy leaves. Take a rug and lie together looking up through the branches of a tree; he'll be fascinated by the play of light and shadow. If this is part of a weekly or daily routine, your baby will learn how the world changes through the seasons, and he'll grow to love his environment. For more adventure, try camping or green festivals (check out the compost port-a-pots and solar-powered showers).

If there's nowhere nice to walk, consider joining a campaign to transform a neglected space like a vacant lot or an old industrial site into an oasis for wildlife. Or start a campaign to plant trees: each one absorbs one ton of carbon dioxide in its lifetime, improves air quality, and cuts urban heat. If roads are too traffic-choked for you to feel safe, protest with other parents by holding a "baby bloc" (read all about it online).

Going for a picnic will introduce your baby to the pleasures of enjoying food in the open air.

Car solutions

Downsizing your car use, or even giving up your car entirely, is perhaps the greenest measure you can take on your baby's behalf.

Cars begin to pollute the environment long before they hit the road; a quarter of the pollutants are thought to be released in the manufacturing process, and the effects hang around long after they've been dumped—in toxic fluids, batteries, tires, plastics, and heavy metals—while the construction of roads endangers habitats, biodiversity, and the water table.

Do biofuels allow greener motoring? Though better for air quality, plant-based fuels are not benign. In northern climates, large-scale cultivation of plants to create bio-ethanol may require as many, or more, fossil fuels than regular fuel (for fertilizers, processing, and transportation). This also ties up agricultural land, perhaps resulting in more air-freighted food. In tropical regions, biofuels are blamed for the clearing of carbon-absorbing forests and for making staple foods, like corn, unaffordable.

To cut emissions and fuel use, first check your tire pressure and remove unnecessary roof racks or weight from the trunk. Keep the windows closed and don't brake suddenly or make jack-rabbit starts. Emissions are lowest at 50 mph and highest over 70 mph. To reduce carbon emissions by 10 percent, switch off the air con—and the engine if stationary for 2 minutes or more.

light green Downsize to a smaller, less-polluting, fuel-efficient car; check the environmental impact of your chosen model on the US Department of Energy's fuel economy website (see p.185). Why not manage with one car, or consider an electric car? Try to go car-free one day a week, or lower the mileage restrictions on your car lease or insurance to make you think twice about hitting the road.

mid green Join a ride-sharing program: each carpool vehicle replaces up to five privately owned cars. Or share a car informally with another family (perhaps instead of a second car). This cuts the cost of maintenance and insurance. Look up the emissions you puff out on each journey on a travel calculator website as a motivation to keep trips to a minimum.

dark green Get rid of your car: in Montreal on Car-Free Day 2004, there was a 90 percent drop in nitrogen monoxide and 100 percent drop in carbon monoxide. This may be tricky in places without good mass transit, and costly (fuel and motoring prices don't reflect environmental costs), but kids whose parents use alternatives to cars are likely to be less car-dependent, more active, and healthier.

ENVIRONMENTAL TOXINS

When you're out and about with your baby, reassure yourself that environmental pollutants can be many times less concentrated outdoors than inside the home.

In a traffic jam, **air pollution** is **3x higher in the car** than on the sidewalk

Each year, some 70,000 different chemicals are released into the environment, many by industry and farming. We are exposed to them wherever and however we live, and not only when we venture outdoors. They are in the air we breathe, the food we eat (or the toys we suck), the water we drink, and the consumer goods we choose. Babies are uniquely vulnerable to the effects of some chemicals in the atmosphere because their cell walls are more permeable than adults'; their nervous, immune, and reproductive systems are still developing; and their detox organs (the liver and kidneys) are not fully functioning.

Hormone-disrupting chemicals in the environment are worrisome because they have the ability to scramble our hormone-regulating system. Even trace levels of the most toxic—known as POPs (persistent organic pollutants)—are harmful, especially to infants, and have been linked with reproductive, behavioral, and immunity problems, and cancer. They are found in everything from fire retardants in furniture and electronics to food, cosmetics, textile finishes, stain protectors, car interiors, nonstick pans, athletic shoes, carpets, and plastic wrap. Need a glass of water? Alongside hormone-disrupting chemicals, it might contain deadly heavy metals and nitrates that reduce the ability of hemoglobin in blood to carry oxygen. Take a deep breath, but not too deep; particulates and PAHs (polycyclic aromatic hydrocarbons, air pollutants created in combustion) from car and heating fumes and cigarette smoke, threaten city dwellers especially. But don't panic; exposure is a fact of modern life, and you can take steps to minimize the risks to your baby. Do get angry enough to write to your representatives and join an environmental organization that campaigns on the issue.

How to reduce your baby's exposure

- Install a water filter.
- Only use certified organic toiletries; your baby doesn't need any bodycare products until he's ready for toothpaste.
- Use eco washing and cleaning products.
- Walk, don't drive: air pollution is higher within a car than outside it during peak travel times.
- Eat organic and dress secondhand.
- Don't smoke: babies exposed to PAHs and smoke have more breathing problems and asthma diagnoses.

Out and about: Green places to go

STAYING SAFE IN THE SUN

A baby's skin is five times thinner than an adult's skin and doesn't yet have a fully developed outer protective layer, so make sure you keep your baby covered up in the sun.

The best coverup is not a chemical sunscreen—even an organic formulation. Insufficient research has been done into the safety of long-term use of sunscreen on young children (even though some daycares won't accept children in summer unless they are wearing sunscreen). Probably the least worrying product is a sunblock, which usually contains ingredients such as zinc or titanium dioxide that sit on the skin's surface, deflecting harmful UV rays. These types of products usually tinge the skin white. Sunscreens are different because they are made from chemical "sponges" that absorb the sun's UV rays and penetrate the skin—and thus don't turn it white. According to the US Environmental Working Group, most sunscreens contain suspect ingredients, such as hormone-disrupting parabens and PABA. If a sunblock or sunscreen boasts that it contains nano ingredients—tiny particles of chemicals—it's probably best to avoid it, since these molecules are so small they may be able to enter the bloodstream; the effects of this are unknown.

    A wide-brimmed hat and coverup clothing are a better choice than sunscreen. Choose lightweight clothes in natural, breathable fabrics with long sleeves or pants. Hemp is a

Keep babies out of direct sunlight and dress them in light, long-sleeved tops, pants, and a hat.

naturally UV-resistant fabric. As an extra precaution, fill your child's plate with sun-protective fruit and vegetables (they tend to be naturally red, orange, or yellow in color). Use a sunshade on your stroller and plan outdoor play sessions for times when the sun is less strong: before 11 am and after 4 pm.

TRAVELING FARTHER AFIELD

Plane journeys are the world's fastest-growing source of CO_2 emissions—and also a nightmare with a wriggly baby on your lap. So what are the greener and easier options for getting away?

Counterintuitively, planes tend to emit fewer greenhouse gases per person than cars—especially if you drive a gas-guzzling SUV. And some journeys on a full, less polluting plane may be more carbon-efficient than driving the same distance by car. The problem is that planes generally travel much greater distances than cars, magnifying the carbon emissions. A single transatlantic flight, for instance, uses more carbon than a whole year's driving in an average car. Planes also deposit warming agents (not just carbon dioxide, but nitrogen and vapor trails) into the atmosphere at high altitude, which may greatly increase their warming impact.

If you are planning to carbon-offset your journey (funding tree-planting or environmental projects in developing countries), do some research first. Companies offering the service are unregulated, the effects of their projects may be hard to verify, or in the case of tree-planting, the environmental benefits are decades away. It may be better to reduce your emissions by insulating your attic, or avoid them completely by not taking that flight. Greener alternatives to the plane are all pretty stressful with a baby or toddler. A train journey may be nine

When you pay for an offset you're not actually neutralizing your carbon impact

times more carbon-efficient than a plane trip, but is limited in terms of baby entertainment. Electric trains are the most carbon-light option.

Long-distance buses can be a greener way to get places, especially if they run on biodiesel or hydrogen fuel cells. But hours of jiggling a restless baby and holding her to the window to take in the view can be tiresome. Ferries can be a more fun way to travel slowly: you can find crawling space and a high-chair, endure a toddler play area or child entertainer, or perhaps even go for a swim. If you book a private cabin, you can even keep to your baby's regular pattern of naps. However, some ferries emit more carbon dioxide than planes, especially high-speed ferries.

The greenest plan is to travel less often. Can you cut your quota to two flights (one round trip)? Having a baby makes you ponder every part of life, so maybe it's time to rethink how frequently you take weekend breaks or long-haul flights.

Conclusion

Now that you've started to change your own life to make it greener, why not spread the word to family, friends, and beyond? Having the support of others really helps to counter green fatigue.

What you can do

- Ask for wooden toys at gift-giving occasions.
- Spread the word that your baby only wears organic or fair-trade clothing.
- Become a breastfeeding counselor.
- Talk your child's playgroup or daycare into using eco cleaning products or switching to a green energy supplier— join the committee to influence which toys and food they buy.
- Involve everyone who cares for your child in your green lifestyle, from nannies to grannies.
- Teach younger family members the basics of home cooking.
- Throw a baby and toddler party in a local park and invite all the children on your street.

We can only make the world a greener place if we act together

Green resources

Campaigning organizations

healthandenvironment.org
The Collaborative on Health and the Environment: organization that works to address growing concerns about the links between human health and environmental factors.

www.foe.org
Friends of the Earth: explore climate change and support campaigns.

www.greenpeace.org
Greenpeace: join campaigns to defend habitats and eliminate toxic chemicals.

www.organicconsumers.org
Organic Consumers Association: nonprofit organization campaigning for health, justice, and sustainability; addresses food safety, genetic engineering, and other key issues.

www.ewg.org
US Environmental Working Group: exposes threats to health and the environment; how to take action.

www.panda.org
WWF (World Wildlife Fund): fight "human-induced" change to the planet.

Health

www.dienviro.com
The Deirdre Imus Environmental Center for Pediatric Oncology: hospital-based program whose aim is to identify, control, and ultimately prevent exposure to environmental factors that may cause cancer, as well as other pediatric health problems.

www.mailman.hs.columbia.edu/ccceh/pollution.html
Columbia Center for Children's Environmental Health: research on the effects of pollution and contaminants.

www.healthychild.org
Healthy Child Healthy World (formerly CHEC): what's harmful for babies; tour a chemical-free home.

www.integrativepeds.org
The Integrative Pediatrics Counsel: aims to increase understanding of the value of integrative healthcare and serve as a resource for those interested in integrative pediatrics.

www.teleosis.org
The Teleosis Institute: organization devoted to developing effective, sustainable healthcare.

www.epa.gov
US Environmental Protection Agency: find out why chemicals in household cleaners can be harmful.

Energy-saving

www.carbonfund.org
Carbonfund.org: how to calculate your carbon footprint, and reduce your environmental impact as much as possible.

www.energysavers.gov
EnergySavers.gov: simple ways to reduce your energy use at home.

www.fueleconomy.gov
US Department of Energy's vehicle fuel economy website.

Ethical consuming

www.actionaidusa.org
Action Aid: the "Who Pays?" campaign highlights corporate accountability.

transfairusa.org
TransFair USA: a nonprofit organization, is one of twenty members of Fairtrade Labeling Organizations International (FLO), and the only third-party certifier of fair-trade products in the United States.

www.fsc.org
Forest Stewardship Council: certifies lumber and "forest products" that protect forests and forest-dependent peoples.

www.freecycle.org
The Freecycle Network: global movement of "giving and getting stuff for free."

www.greensage.com
GreenSage: information on sustainable home furnishings and materials.

www.thegreenguide.com
The Green Guide (National Geographic): tips, tools, blogs, and articles on green living.

Green baby goods

www.ecobaby.com
Ecobaby Organics: eco baby goods, plus information on product certification.

www.naturalcollection.com
Natural Collection: online eco department store.

www.realdiaperassociation.org
The Real Diaper Association: call for the nearest source of cloth diapers.

www.purebeginnings.com
Pure Beginnings: baby apparel and bedding made from organic cotton. Also sells natural bath and skincare products for babies.

Green foods

www.allorganiclinks.com
AllOrganicLinks.com: information on sourcing healthy, organic foods.

www.babyledweaning.com
Baby-led Weaning: how to skip pureed food and jump straight to family food.

www.eatwiththeseasons.com
Eating with the Seasons: what's fresh and delicious in your area.

www.lllusa.org
La Leche League: mother-to-mother breastfeeding support and helpline.

www.ams.usda.gov/farmersmarkets
AMS Farmers' Markets: information on how to find a local farmers' market.

www.mbayaq.org/cr/SeafoodWatch.asp
Monterey Bay Aquarium: guide to healthy, eco-friendly seafood choices.

Green toys

www.kidbean.com
KidBean.com: sells all-natural wooden and organic toys.

Greener travel

www.thebabywearer.com
The Baby Wearer: global reviews of slings and research into "baby-wearing."

www.worldcarfree.net
World Carfree Network: statistics and arguments for giving up your car.

Green resources

Glossary

ACO: Australian Certified Organic.

Antioxidants: molecules that minimize the harmful effects of free radicals, typically found in certain fruit and vegetables.

BDIH: the Federation of German Industries and Trading certifies natural cosmetics as not tested on animals and GM-free; manufacture is eco-friendly.

CE Marking: safety mark certifying the product's conformity to the essential requirements of European law.

Dioxins: dangerous toxins, formed as byproducts of certain manufacturing processes; some are known carcinogens.

Fairtrade: the Fairtrade mark is an independent consumer label which guarantees producers in the developing world are getting a better deal.

Flavonoids: a group of compounds with antioxidant properties (also known as bioflavonoids).

FSC: the Forest Stewardship Council, promotes responsible management of the world's forests.

GM: genetically modified crops or organisms have been altered artificially to produce desirable characteristics.

KRAV: the Swedish body regulating organic standards belongs to the International Federation of Organic Agriculture Movements.

Lion Mark: a consumer safety symbol.

Nonylphenol: a synthetic organic compound, used as an industrial surfactant, but now banned in Europe.

Organotins: tin-based compounds, used industrially as heat stabilizers and as biocides, but highly toxic to marine life.

PABA: para-aminobenzoic acid, used as a filter in sunscreens, but linked to cancer.

PAHs: polycyclic aromatic hydrocarbons, released in combustion, are associated with many dangers to health.

PCBs: polychlorinated biphenyls had various industrial uses, but are now banned and classed as POPs.

Phthalates: compounds used mainly as plasticizers, linked to hormone disruption.

    BBP: butyl benzyl phthalate.

    DBP: di-n-butyl phthalate.

    DEHP: di (2-ethylhexyl) phthalate.

    DIDP: di-isodecyl phthalate.

    DINP: di-isononyl phthalate.

    DNOP: di-n-octyl phthalate.

POPs: persistent organic pollutants.

PVC: polyvinyl chloride is a plastic with very many commercial applications; it is thought to pose significant health risks.

SLS: sodium lauryl sulphate is a surfactant detergent; it is found in the majority of bodycare products, and is associated with various health complaints.

Toluene: a water-insoluble liquid used in industrial products; chronic inhalation can result in brain damage.

US EPA: United States Environmental Protection Agency.

UV: ultraviolet electromagnetic radiation.

VOCs: volatile organic compounds.

Index

Acknowledgments

Author's acknowledgments
The author would like to thank: Ethical Consumer; CAT; Weleda; Greg and Teresa Pascoe at Cusgarne Farm; Paul Slydel at Cycle Solutions (01326 377003); Julia Linfoot BSc MCPH RSHom for text on homeopathic remedies; toxicologist John Marriott; Mary Mathieson; and everyone at DK, especially Penny and Peggy, and above all Tara and Hannah.

Publisher's acknowledgments
Dorling Kindersley would like to thank Sue Bosanko for indexing; Alyson Silverwood for proofreading; Peggy Sadler for design assistance; Andrea Bagg and Diana Vowles for editorial assistance; the following for the loan of props: Yummies (01273 738733), Great Expectations (01273 622993), Greenfibres, Holz Toys, Beaming Baby, Wool Shed (www. woolshed.co.uk), Little Hooligan (www. littlehooligan.com), Bamboo Baby (www. bamboobaby.co.uk), Tatty Bumpkin (www. tattybumpkin.com), By Nature (www. bynature.co.uk), Blackout Kitsch (01273 671741), Hen & Hammock (www. henandhammock.co.uk), Sidney Street Bikes, and Paperpod (www.paperpod.co.uk).
Our models were: Miro & Mina Lloyd, Eleanor & Isabella Moore-Smith, Kitty & Juliette Kinsman, Sarah Coats & Rafael Apey, Louise Rainey & Samuel Pole, Jeya James, Amias Limerick, Elizabeth Apple & Isla Apple Hall, Corrine Ashgar, Oliver & Alex Roberts, Ry Zeferino-Birchall, Amber Asamoa, Ruby Baker, Torsten Van Ande, Meera Vithaldas, Gaia Dean & Mia Beugre, Heather Lewis & Robyn Moody, Nicole Drysdale, John, Ruben & Louis Harrison, Hannah Bellanche, Mattie Barrett, Kevin Smith, Rachael Parfitt & Eddie Hunt.

Picture credits
The publisher would like to thank the following for their kind permission to reproduce their photographs:
(Key: b—bottom; c—center)
Alamy Images: Bubbles Photolibrary 32; Ingram Publishing (Superstock Limited) 69bc; Niall McDiarmid 138; David Pearson 56; Getty Images: Adamsmith 160; John Millar 124; Antonio Mo 11; Greg Pease 16; Chris Rawlings 70; Arthur Tilley 156; iStockphoto.com: UteHil 43; PunchStock: RubberBall 102

All other images © Dorling Kindersley
For further information see:
www.dkimages.com